The
Longevity
Bible

Susannah Marriott

The definitive guide to a long, healthy and happy life

GODSFIELD

For my husband, our girls,
and their grandparents.

An Hachette UK Company
www.hachette.co.uk

First published in Great Britain in 2018 by Godsfield Press,
a division of Octopus Publishing Group Ltd,
Carmelite House,
50 Victoria Embankment, London EC4Y 0DZ
www.octopusbooks.co.uk

Text copyright © Susannah Marriott 2018
Design and layout copyright © Octopus Publishing Group Ltd 2018

ISBN 978-1-84181-475-9

A CIP catalogue record for this book is available from the British Library.

Printed and bound in China
10 9 8 7 6 5 4 3 2 1

All reasonable care has been taken in the preparation of this book, but the information it contains is to be used for educational and information purposes only, and is not intended to take the place of any advice, counselling or treatment given by a qualified practitioner. While all exercises and practices in this book are completely safe if followed correctly, you must consult a specialist before making any changes to your diet, lifestyle or health and fitness regime, and seek professional advice if you have any existing conditions or concerns.

The Publisher disclaims to any person or entity, any liability, loss or damage (alleged or caused), directly or indirectly as a result of the use, application or interpretation of the contents of this book.

Commissioning Editor: Leanne Bryan
Art Director: Yasia Williams-Leedham
Junior Editor: Ella Parsons
Copy Editor: Marion Paull
Designer: Sally Bond
Picture Research Manager: Jennifer Veall
Production Controller: Dasha Miller

Contents

Introduction:
experience, perspective, resilience

What is longevity? The dictionary has it as living to a great age, but there's another meaning – if something has longevity, it has constancy and persistence, for as much as long life itself is great, it's not as useful a goal as a good, abundant and durable life. This book is about what we can do to live better for longer; it's about expanding our "health span" and enhancing wellbeing with each year that passes.

This is not an anti-ageing book. Ageing defines the human condition – we are all ageing all the time, however old we are. Ageing also defines the universal condition. For more than half its 13-something billion years the universe has been ageing, its energy output waning on all frequencies and in all galaxies, the rate at which new stars are made slowing and the temperature of everything cooling. We are connected to time whether we like it or not. To deny that, to strive to be something we're not, somehow ashamed about being or looking our age, to define "successful" ageing by the characteristics of youth is not good for our mental health or wellbeing.

This book is kinder than that. It encourages us to be more generous and authentic. It celebrates all the good of ageing – the wisdom, experience and confidence extra years bring – and offers life-affirming ways to maintain equilibrium and lust for life at any age.

Good ageing is about being increasingly resilient to the stuff life throws at us – change, loss, adversity – so we are able to process it in a way that keeps life feeling meaningful and satisfying, and we remain motivated to bounce back and try new things. What makes us resilient? An active life with a good diet and enough sleep, a sense of life-satisfaction and self-esteem, positive brain stimulation, satisfying human interaction and spiritual sustenance. That's what this book is about. The good news is that resilience doesn't decline with age – older people are at least as resilient as younger adults, studies suggest. It doesn't seem to be affected by where we live, be that in a rural, urban or suburban environment, and it may be even greater if we have a mental illness.

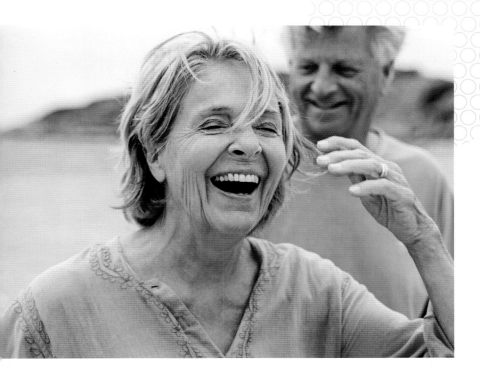

I've included a lot of yoga because I see the benefits in my fellow older yogis and especially our teachers. Yoga is brilliant for physical health as we age (improving bone and muscle strength, coordination, flexibility, breathing and circulation), it keeps the brain active, the mind conscious, promotes relaxation and sleep, and encourages hormonal balance and a positive outlook. It makes us more responsive to changes in body and emotions and raises sensory

ABOVE: At its best, ageing is a time of liberation and exploration that allows us to make the most of every day.

awareness. It's also reputed to tune us in to spiritual powers – wisdom, intuition, clarity of vision – that liberate us from the negativity associated with ageing, disease, even death.

We're looking in on other insightful takes on ageing, especially from Ayurveda, the traditional Indian healthcare system, and Traditional Chinese Medicine (TCM),

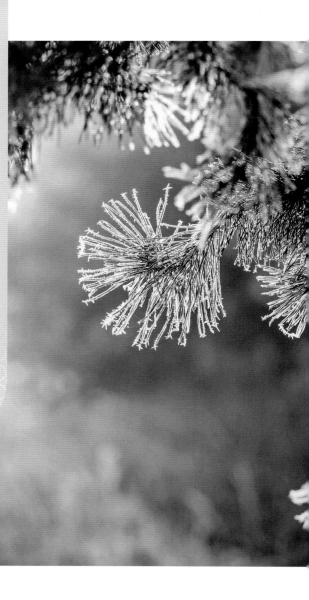

"If at every stage of your life you do the right thing, your actions will bring remarkable dividends when you have lived a long time and achieved a great deal. This is not only because you will never have to second-guess your actions, not even at the supreme moment, at the very end of life, but because of the great pleasure that comes from looking back on a long life well-spent and on many deeds well done."

CICERO

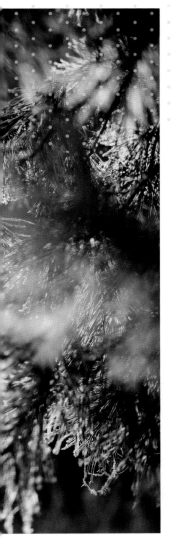

and at archetypal stories and fables that help us come to terms with some of the darker sides of ageing. Tales of going into the underworld or setting out on a quest for eternal life express our deepest fears and hopes, while symbols of ageing done well, such as the tortoise, pine and winter (see pages 288, 251 and 384), can feel incredibly resonant.

This is a book full of hope and possibilities that bears testament to our potential for lifelong learning and dynamic transformation.

LEFT: In the beauty of winter we can contemplate the best qualities of older age: a stillness and deep rest that nourish creative energy.

NON-NEGOTIABLES WE NEED TO AGE WELL

- Plenty of exercise
- Nourishing food
- Good rest
- Better breathing
- Calm and focused mind
- Brain food
- Kind community
- Friends of all ages
- Joyful spirit
- Strength to withstand storms

The state of age we're in

Over the past one hundred years life expectancy has been growing steadily and continually; the World Health Organization (WHO) calls it one of the 20th century's greatest achievements.

That's thanks to improvements in our environment – water, diet, air quality – and because we vaccinate children against infectious diseases. Better nourishment and exposure to fewer diseases in childhood mean many more of us survive and thrive.

We've been growing older slower in the past few decades in particular, due to more people having given up smoking, improvements in the treatment of heart disease and cancer, and increased child survival and HIV treatment in Africa. The average life span has increased dramatically in the 21st century: between 2000 and 2015 average life expectancy around the globe increased by five years, the fastest since the 1960s, says the WHO, fastest of all in Africa. Global

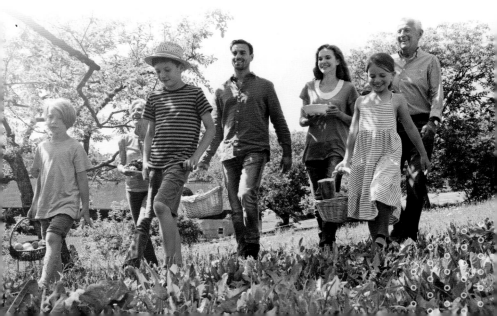

life expectancy is now at 73.8 years for women and 69.1 for men, set to rise to 85.3 and 78.1 by 2030. Japan is the world leader, at more than 83 years, but everywhere is seeing an improvement in life expectancy for the over-80s. Regardless of changes in life span, the gender gap stays the same: according to data from the United Nations, women live around 4.5 years longer than men.

In Australia, as elsewhere, the baby-boomer generation has been getting older, meaning the number of people at retirement age has been increasing rapidly. In the US, the number of people aged over 85 is set to more than triple by 2060. And in the UK, The Office of National Statistics predicts that around 22 per cent of the population will be 65-plus by 2031 (outnumbering under-25s). However, there's been an unanticipated stalling of late in England and Wales – mortality improvement is flattening off and we don't know why. Some say we've reaped the benefits of quitting smoking and the more effective treatment of heart disease; others say this is a result of the austerity cuts following the economic crash of 2008.

In key places around the world, known as Blue Zones, longevity is particularly marked, and astoundingly high numbers

of centenarians are living active, happy lives into their second century. On the Mediterranean islands of Sardinia and Icaria, the Japanese islands of Okinawa, on the Costa Rican Nicoya Peninsula and in the Seventh Day Adventist community of Loma Linda in California, common lifestyle factors give clues to what makes for a long and fulfilling old age largely free from the conditions of ageing, such as heart disease and cataracts. They are really quite obvious and simple things – lifelong physical activity, a diet rich in plant foods, a clean environment, sustaining spiritual life, a purposeful role and a supportive community that makes room for rest and values its elders as custodians of tradition.

We've mythologized these places, likening them to the mythical Greek isle of Hyperborea, a distant land "beyond the north wind" where there is perpetual spring and the inhabitants live for a thousand years, free of disease, old age and war. When they wish to end their lives, they leap into a lake and are transformed into white swans. The people of the Blue Zone Shangri-Las prove that our biological age doesn't have to match our chronological age.

> **TIP:** Find out how old your body actually is by searching for a "What's My Biological Age?" online quiz.

LEFT: Life expectancy has increased with each generation – and in every country throughout the world – over the past 200 years.

How we age

Physiologically, the body deteriorates with the wear and tear of time. Even if they stay healthy, all our body systems are affected by age. In evolutionary terms, we're primed to pass on our genes in the reproductive decades and then head into decline.

The ageing process speeds markedly after our fertile years. Heart rate and output and volume of blood all decrease while the arteries harden and blood pressure increases; the lungs don't exchange gas as effectively and drop in capacity. Heart disease, stroke and pulmonary disease claim most lives around the globe, accounting for around a third of all deaths. Heart disease is the leading cause of mortality as we hit 65.

Since most of us stop being so active as we age, muscle cells atrophy and bone and lean body mass reduce; we lose muscle power and endurance and our range of movement and flexibility declines. Joints degenerate. The gastrointestinal system slows along with our metabolism. Hormone production ebbs, immunity reduces, inflammation becomes more likely.

The brain shrinks physically and becomes slower at processing and problem-solving; the memory falters and senses fade. Alzheimer's, the most common form of dementia, is the fifth leading cause of death globally, above road injuries, HIV/AIDS and diabetes. Cases almost double every five years after the age of 65 – while fewer than 3 per cent of people in their late 60s have it, almost 30 per cent of the over-85s do.

Past generations tended to die from infectious and parasitic diseases – smallpox, polio, measles – associated with poor diet and environment. Now the leading causes of death are non-communicable and chronic conditions, such as heart disease, cancer and diabetes. According to the WHO, these represent 87 per cent of disease in people over 60. However, there's tremendous individual variability in both the onset of ageing and the age at which we contract these diseases.

Why we age

Research into the genetic make-up of long-lived people has identified which genes are involved and where they mutate to affect our life span (the age-1 gene). Sibling and geographical studies have looked at the balance of environment to genetic heritage in the ageing process.

YOUNG AT HEART

It's a phenomenon remarked on through the ages that very old people commonly report that they don't feel old inside, and don't identify as old, whatever the age they reach. This seems to correlate in the English Longitudinal Study of Ageing with increased life expectancy. The essentials that make us feel vital are age-irrelevant – a stable and supple body, peaceful focused mind and harmonious spirit. As German writer and philosopher Goethe noted, "Age takes hold of us by surprise."

The world's oldest person ever certainly didn't feel her age. This supercentenarian, Jeanne Calment from Arles in France, lived to 122 years 164 days, finally leaving us in 1997. She remembered meeting Van Gogh in her home town and seeing the Eiffel Tower being built. Jeanne took up fencing at 85 and practised both gymnastics and piano until she was 109. Her record is as much a testament to the quality of French record-keeping and population registration as it is to her youthful spirit and good health.

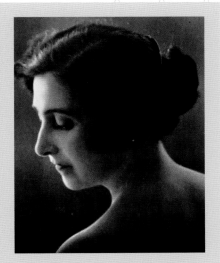

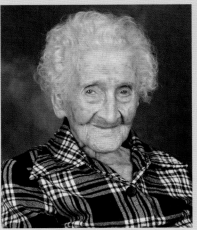

ABOVE: Jeanne Calment, offically the world's oldest person yet recorded, in her youth and healthy old age.

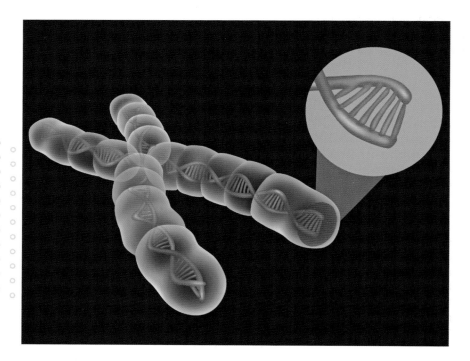

It seems that 20–30 per cent of the variation in how we age is due to genetics, and that this is more important in men than women; the older you get, the more the genetic factor kicks in.

DNA and telomeres

We don't yet understand all the body processes that contribute to ageing, but we do know it's important to keep the DNA in cells protected from harm, because we age when our DNA is

ABOVE: The DNA inside the chromosome is protected at its end by the telomere (coloured here in red).

damaged. All cells have a life span – they can divide only so many times, and the number of divisions declines as we age. Newborn cells divide 80–90 times when cultured in labs; those from a 70-year-old around 20–30 times. When cells stop being able to divide, they function less efficiently, then die. That may contribute to the slowing in wound-healing as the decades pass and to reduced immunity and the build-up of atherosclerosis in damaged blood-vessel walls.

The number of healthy divisions may be determined by the protective casing at the end of genes, telomeres. These are "repetitive" lengths of DNA and proteins that stabilize the ends of chromosomes. Every time a cell divides the telomere shortens because the cell can't replicate DNA well at the ends of a strand, so older organisms tend to have shorter telomeres. When the telomere gets too short, the cell can't divide any more and dies (cell "senescence"). An enzyme called telomerase counters this shortening by repairing and replenishing the length of the telomeres, but our supply decreases with age and chronic stress, especially stress connected with adverse life circumstances and depression.

There's an association between shortened telomeres and some of the key health conditions of ageing – osteoporosis, heart disease, diabetes – as well as worsened functioning of the organs and atrophying tissue. Longer telomeres are associated with decreased development of age-related disease.

However, conflicting research studies show that mice with healthily long telomeres don't live longer, and that cancer cells activate telomerase, which in turn strengthens the telomeres, with the result that the cancerous cells become immortal. Furthermore, cells can divide many more times than required for a human life span. Something else must be at work in the ageing process.

Mitochondria

Each of our cells contains mitochondria, power-generators that absorb and break down nutrients and release around 90 per cent of the chemical energy a cell needs to stay active and alive. Muscle cells, such as brain and heart cells, in particular, need lots of energy so contain many thousands of mitochondria. These power-pack "organelles" also play a role in breaking down and recycling waste, and in triggering cell death. With age, performance of the mitochondrial network declines, as free-radical damage (see page 16) and mutation impair its function. This is linked to a weakening in muscle, brain and heart cells in particular, and can play a role in common diseases of ageing.

INTRODUCTION

Researchers at institutions including the École Polytechnique Fédérale de Lausanne, Switzerland, and University of California, Berkley have found that reducing the output of mitochondria early in life – by exposing them to mild stress – can lead to an increase in efficiency of the mitochondria in mice and nematode worms throughout life, boosting the metabolism and life span of these creatures. Investigations at Harvard Chan School of Public Health found that restricting the diet of nematode worms seemed to keep the mitochondrial networks youthful. The next stage is to carry out tests on mammals. In the meantime, we can keep the body stimulated to delay mitochondrial ageing and trigger the creation of new mitochondria ("biogenesis") with regular exercise, good sleep and eating a diet rich in healthy fats and vegetables.

Oxidative damage

Cellular ageing may result from oxidative damage. Free radicals (the product of electrons combining with oxygen molecules), created as a by-product of cellular processes and in response to UV light and air pollution, damage the mitochondria in cells. Oxidative stress has been linked with ageing of the brain in particular and with cataracts and cancer.

The free-radical theory of ageing dates from the 1950s, based on the observation that oxidative damage increases with age, and that reducing oxidative damage extends the life span of fruit flies, mice and other lab-test species. (Antioxidants spare our cells from the effects of free radicals by becoming oxidized themselves.) But an increasing number of studies have found that increased antioxidant production can shorten life and that ageing happens even in anaerobic conditions (without oxygen).

More to discover

Oxidative damage seems to be just one of many forms of damage from our many biological processes, all of which contribute to ageing. We can work out how to fix one form of damage, but because we are a mass of interconnected systems and parts, that can cause another part of the whole to misfire. We are biologically imperfect, say the researchers, and can't predict outcomes – that may be the true cause of ageing in the end. That and random other factors we don't yet understand.

AYURVEDA AND AGEING

The traditional Indian healthcare system considers itself a "science" of long life. It regards everything in the universe, including our bodies, to be made up of the same basic elements: earth, water, fire, air and ether. When they are in equilibrium, we are strong and live long. We maintain balance by living according to the seasons and with "good conduct", developing a healthy daily routine and eating a diet rich in rejuvenating foods and herbal preparations, and by cultivating a lifestyle sympathetic to our individual constitution.

Ayurveda sees the body as a mix of three *doshas*, or constitutional energies – *vata*, *pitta* and *kapha*. *Vata* is an airy energy, an active force that controls all movement, from breathing to blood flow, as well as nerves and electronic impulses. *Pitta* is the body's inner fire, and oversees metabolism, the endocrine system and digestion. *Kapha* is the heavy grounding force that structures the body in space, manifesting in connective tissue and mucus. When one *dosha* becomes over-dominant, the health of the whole is affected – too much dry, airy *vata* might manifest as osteoporosis or arthritis; too much *pitta* heat as high

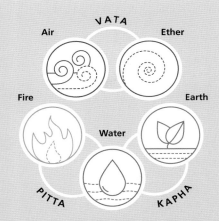

ABOVE: The three *doshas* that make up our Ayurvedic constitution are formed from the elements earth, water, fire, air and ether.

blood pressure or flushes; too much cold, heavy *kapha* as constipation or oedema.

Different *doshas* come to the fore in various life stages, manifesting in the ailments of that era. *Kapha* predominates in childhood, gradually shifting to *pitta* in our 40s and 50s, shown in symptoms such as hot flushes. After about 55 we have more *vata*, seen in the disintegration of bones and memory. We are encouraged to adopt *vata*-reducing strategies (see page 336) in the later decades to combat the conditions associated with ageing.

TRADITIONAL CHINESE MEDICINE AND AGEING

The Chinese system of "internal alchemy" says the more we have of the Three Treasures, the more we ensure longevity, and urges us to work to keep them balanced. They are *qi* (life force, see page 334), *jing* (vital essence, see page 247) and *shen* (spiritual energy, see page 349). We bring the three into balance by practising tai chi or qigong, which leads to vigour, stamina and strength as well as ease of movement in body and mind.

It's said we are born with a finite amount of *jing*, the primal force responsible for the developmental process from birth through growth to decline and death. It protects us from the onslaught of the six key factors thought to cause disease: summer heat, dryness, damp, cold, heat (fire) and wind. *Jing* determines our strength and resilience, and the more we maintain a good store, the longer we live. It represents our genetic make-up and can't be topped up (unlike *qi*).

Jing is stored in the kidneys (it's also known as kidney essence) and powers us as we grow into adulthood, peaking around our early 20s and fuelling the creation of new life. As we head past 40 the energy naturally depletes (from the upper body first). We weaken physically and become more prone to disease – all symptoms diminish *jing*, leaving us even more depleted and vulnerable. Chronic stress is especially depleting. Death results when there is no more *jing*.

In order to minimize the amount of *jing* we "leak", we are recommended to adopt a healthy diet, relieve stress with sleep, exercise, relaxation and meditation, take tonic herbs (see page 246) and strengthen the kidney meridian through acupuncture and by practising tai chi or qigong.

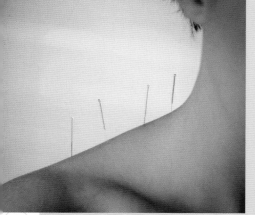

LEFT: Traditional Chinese Medicine advocates techniques that work on the meridians – subtle energy channels – to maintain health as we age.

The stages of life

Throughout history we've come up with a recipe for living that divides our life span into neatly defined chapters, each with a code of behaviour befitting that life stage, and lessons that help us progress to the next rung.

It's a "hero's journey"; in each act, we learn something that allows us to move forward and become more whole, until at the end of life we stand transformed. These stages may reveal themselves only in retrospect.

Each stage has its season, Cicero wrote, and its defining quality – seriousness in adulthood and maturity in older age – suggesting this is a fixed and natural path. In the ancient Greek era, man (and it was men) passed from the prime of life as warriors into the affairs of state, wisdom learned in battle fitting them to pass judgment and make decisions for a community.

The earliest depiction of the stages of life can be detected in a blackened fresco in the desert castle of Qasr Amra, Jordan. There are three stages here. The earliest forms of worship are of the triple-goddess, a woman in the three phases of her reproductive life, maiden, mother and crone, often compared to the phases of the moon, waxing, full and waning. Crone qualities that older women may

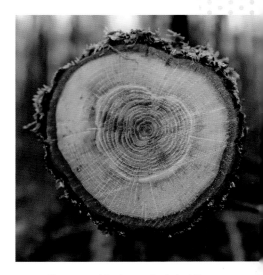

ABOVE: The passage of time is most pleasingly visible in the concentric rings of a tree's growth, where we can read the story of each year's weather.

find empowering include the wisdom and patience, perspective and generosity gained through experience, often on journeys through life's dark times. The Greek crone goddess Hecate (see page 150) understands and can wield the powers of the underworld – including divination and intuition – to do good. She speaks the truth and brings riches and victory.

The stages-of-life trope speaks loudest in medieval Europe. Here, there are most often four stages – childhood, youth, adulthood and old age – analogous to the four elements, seasons and cardinal points (our earliest symbolic and magical preoccupations). In the Hindu tradition, too, life is a path of four stages or *ashrama*. *Brahmacharya*, the student stage, is for learning and preparation. At *Grihastha*, householder stage, we are busy with family and jobs, focused in the world. At 50, *Vanaprastha* begins, the "hermit" stage at which we start to disengage from home and work preoccupations and are urged to retreat to the forest for contemplation. The final stage, *Sannyasa*, wandering, is one of total renunciation – of possessions and responsibilities – to focus on self-realization in preparation for rebirth.

Sometimes there are seven stages of life – in Shakespeare's famous seven ages of man monologue ("All the world's a stage" from *As You Like It*), the seven stages correspond to qualities ascribed to the planets in the ancient world, and the order in which they orbit earth: the moon represents childhood, Mercury the scholarly years, Venus the time of forming relationships and homes, Mars the soldier marching out to make a mark on the world, Jupiter the time of justice and rule, with Saturn for old age, the slowest-moving of the planets, considered the great teacher in astrology. As the

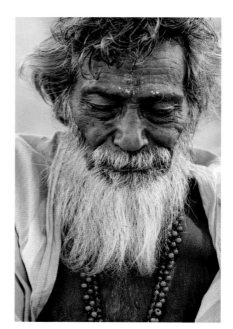

RIGHT: A Hindu *sannyasi* renounces the material world and family ties in order to pursue devotional practices and a spiritual life.

most distant star, Saturn is associated with the limits of awareness. There is no planet allocated to the very oldest years in Shakespeare's monologue. It is "mere oblivion, sans teeth, sans eyes, sans taste, sans everything". For beyond Saturn was the unknown realm of the stars.

Seven is a number often used in connection with the stages of life, chiming with sacred timescales: the seven days of creation, the days of the week named for the Norse and Germanic gods and the planets of the classical world. Solon in 6th-century Greece recognized ten seven-year cycles, each bringing a different aspect to maturity: mind and ethics at 42, skills in speaking and thinking between 49 and 56. Pythagoras considered multiples of seven – 21, 49, 56, 63 – to be especially significant life-markers, and announced that old age started at 60.

Increasingly today we're encouraged to think beyond chronological definitions of age. We are old not at 60 or 80 but at the point at which body and mind no longer serve our desires and allow us agency.

WISE WOMEN AGEING

Traditional Chinese Medicine sees women's lives as rolling out in seven seven-year cycles. This was first described in the *Yellow Emperor's Classic of Internal Medicine*, the oldest known document in Chinese Medicine, which probably dates from around 300 BCE. These seven-year cycles account for the reproductive years only, ending at age 49, when conception is said to become unlikely. Seven is an odd number, considered *yin* to the male eight-year *yang* cycle.

But women continue to evolve in seven-year cycles throughout life, suggests psychoanalyst and poet Dr Clarissa Pinkola Estés, author of the classic work *Women Who Run With the Wolves*. With each cycle we become more aware of how the world works and more aligned with the spiritual life, she argues, her series of seven-year cycles spooling out beyond the age of 105.

The loss of the monthly cycle around which our reproductive life revolves can leave women feeling untethered and lacking in focus. We can re-orient ourselves and create a continuing sense of order or progress by watching the rotations of the moon throughout the month. We might feel more expansive as it waxes, and draw into ourselves and look within as it wanes, resting more at the full and new moons. Each month's new moon brings a new opportunity to refocus and take stock.

Extending life – fact and fiction

The steady rise in life expectancy – about three months per year between 1840 and 2007, says the WHO – raises the question of our potential life span. Does it even have an upper limit? Scientists are investigating this right now, but artists, writers and philosophers have always been curious about the fountain of life eternal, and what follows if we drink from it.

Some scientists dispute that we have a biological clock that runs out at a certain point. If we can understand the causes of ageing, they say, it could be possible to delay its negative effects in perpetuity. In 2017 five research teams writing in the journal *Nature* refuted a claim from the International Database on Longevity (which tracks supercentenarians around the globe) that the human age-ceiling has plateaued at 114.9 years since the mid-1990s. They point at studies predicting a life span of 150 years by 2300 and call this stalling a mere blip (a single cold winter in decades of global warming).

The current generation of supercentenarians (people verifiably aged 110 or over) are subject to huge research interest. Centenarians tend to stay markedly healthy, delay the onset of common age-related disease and live independently into their 90s. Supercentenarians are the healthiest of the lot – the older you get, the healthier you've been. The good news is that people who live for an exceptionally long time tend to lead long and healthy lives regardless of genetics or of social or cultural background. Any serious illness is crammed into a few years at the very end of life ("compressed morbidity").

CLASSIFYING THE VERY OLD

The New England Centenarian Study classifies the centenarians they study in the following categories of health:

- **Escapers** – no signs of disease at age 100 (15 per cent of people studied)
- **Delayers** – no signs of disease until 80 or later (43 per cent of people studied)
- **Survivors** – age-related disease diagnosed before 80 (42 per cent of people studied)

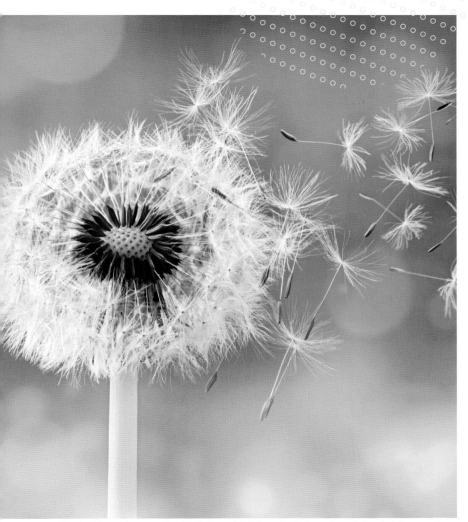

ABOVE: The dandelion, perhaps more beautiful in its aged state than when in flower, is a potent symbol of regeneration: a single plant produces some 15,000 new seeds.

What does the supercentenarian cohort tell us about longevity? According to the New England Centenarian Study, if you are a man and live past 100 you are 17 times more likely than a "regular" person to have siblings also over 100, and your kids, aged 65-plus, will experience substantially delayed diseases of ageing, such as cardiovascular disease, diabetes and "overall mortality". Some families are markedly long-lived and investigators are looking at their DNA to try to isolate key genes, in particular the insulin-pathway gene, genes related to cholesterol metabolism and those linked with lower incidence of high-blood pressure, cardiovascular disease and memory loss.

The fact of being a woman seems to be a genetic advantage in itself – figures from the Office for National Statistics show that 85 per cent of centenarians and around 90 per cent of supercents are women. The few men are very healthy, though – women seem better at living with age-related disease (it's not known why) whereas men who live to a great age are just healthier throughout life.

We all have the potential to hit our late 80s in great shape if we look after ourselves, advises the New England Centenarian Study, after following the largest number of supercentenarians of any research. After this point, it's all about genetic factors, and the race for the genetic key to infinity is on.

COMMON CHARACTERISTICS OF CENTENARIANS

The New England Centenarian Study notes these characteristics common to a study-group diverse in ethnicity, wealth, education and diet:

• Lean bodyweight

• Unlikely to have smoked

• Good at handling stress

• Healthy brains

• Gave birth post-40 (a sign the body is ageing slowly)

• Very old siblings and very healthy children

The quest for eternal life

The resurrection myth has been with us from the beginning – we observe the turning seasons and crave reassurance that after the bleakness of winter, the sun will return and there will be new growth to sustain us.

One of its earliest expressions is in Ishtar, Babylonian goddess of life and fertility (aka the Sumerian Inanna). She appears in the world's oldest written story, the *Epic of Gilgamesh*, and is remembered for her quest to conquer the underworld. She is put to death but revived, and returns to the world on condition her husband takes her place in the underworld for half the year. Her story is reborn in the tale of Persephone (see page 382).

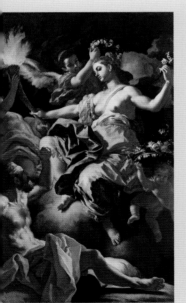

BE CAREFUL WHAT YOU WISH FOR

The ancient Greeks warned of the perils of anti-ageing. Overwhelmed with love for her mortal husband, the young and beautiful winged goddess of the day, Eos (aka Aurora – she rides Pegasus), begs Zeus to make him live forever. He consents, but withholds the corresponding gift of eternal youth. Eos watches her lover's slow decline from handsome hunk to weak old man – she feeds him "celestial ambrosia", the drink of the gods that confers immortality and supposedly preserves mortal flesh, but mortals who take it never thrive. When, finally, he becomes too decrepit for movement or thought, she locks him away. Eventually the gods take pity and turn him into a cicada. We can hear him still today, begging for release from life. Immortality is too much for mortals to bear.

LEFT: As dawn breaks, the light of immortal Aurora dazzles the weak eyes of her mortal husband Tithonus, who ages with each new day.

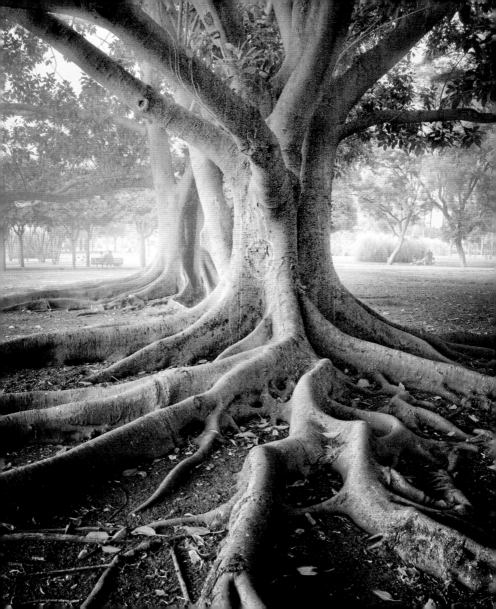

At the foot of the Tree of Life in the Christian and Islamic depiction of Paradise springs a fountain, the pure waters of which flow out to the four cardinal points, similar to the Fountain of Memory at the entrance to the Greek underworld. Drinking from it guarantees immortality. Ever-living waters spout most profusely in the 15th century, when heroes of romances discover lakes of youthfulness and paintings depict old women diving in to emerge as beautiful young things. The fountain of youth, emblem of untold riches, was reputed to be in a jungle in the New World, and in 1513 Spanish conquistador Juan Ponce de Léon set off to find it, so they said after his death. He "discovered" Florida instead, and we can drink the healing waters in St Augustine still.

LEFT: Ancient trees have ancient roots, and are a common feature of foundation myths the world over.

Is it in the blood?

If not water, then is blood the antidote to ageing? The Bible tells us "the life of a creature is in the blood" (Leviticus 17:11), and in the sacrament of communion it is the blood of Christ that offers remission of sins and life eternal. Ovid in his *Metamorphosis* describes the enchantress Medea bringing Jason's elderly father back to life by letting his own blood and replacing it with a rich elixir that turns his white hair dark and lustrous and renews youthful vigour to his wasted form. There are many early-modern descriptions of the blood of young people being used to restore old men to health – pour it in "as if from the fountain of life," advised chemist Andreas Libavius in 1616, "and all of his weaknesses will be dispelled."

IMMORTALITY SCIENCE FICTION

Writers and artists have always been drawn to the notion of perpetual life. An entire sub-genre of speculative fiction known as "immortality science fiction" is addressing questions prompted by the longevity scientists: would eternal life be available for everyone, what would we have to give up in return, and how would we tolerate eons of history? If no one can die, are there wars, and what is the ultimate sacrifice? When does human life stop and Artificial Intelligence (AI) start? The creatures of popular culture who do live forever – zombies, vampires, the undead – don't seem especially happy in their immortal state; and there's a grisly warning in the 1965 Hammer film *She* based on H Rider Haggard's novel, in which immortal queen Ayesha, played by Ursula Andress, ages millennia in seconds.

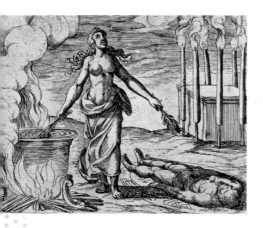

Technology and ageing

The fountain of youth as a source of never-ending riches is still turning base materials to gold. Solving the problem of death is the new quest of some of the world's most powerful companies. The moguls behind Google, Amazon, Apple and PayPal are putting massive investment into labs, biotech startups and foundations to "cure" ageing with new tools – machine learning, algorithms, artificial intelligence (AI) and methodologies used to hack and crack code. There are programmes on "geroprotection" to predict our expiry date by pinpointing and tracking the biomarkers of ageing, on growth-hormone and stem-cell therapy and gene editing, on growing DNA-personalized organs, transhumanism (merging with other species) and downloading memories so part of us does live forever – in mechanical form or on the cloud. Then there is Facebook's Mark Zuckerberg and wife Priscilla Chan's mission to "cure all disease".

Inspired by the Medea story, people were experimenting with animal-to-animal transfusion from around 1639 (in England on chickens). In the first successful transfusion of life in 1665, Cornish doctor Richard Lower proved a dog could be brought to the point of death by loss of blood, then restored to life with another dog's blood.

Young blood for new life is still a thing – after trials showed that putting young blood into old mice reversed cognitive and neurological impairment, Californian startup Ambrosia (note the name) launched a crowdfunded trial recruiting 600 people of median age 60 (at $8,000 a pop) to receive plasma from 16–25-year-olds. There's no good evidence to link the treatment with anti-ageing effects, either in mice or humans.

These quests circumvent and disrupt conventional medical research. America's Food and Drug Administration (FDA) and other world authorities that regulate drugs and their funding don't recognize ageing as a disease, and biological substances such as plasma can't be patented and sold.

IN SEARCH OF A MAGIC FORMULA

There's often something to give in exchange for eternal youth – most famously a deal with the devil. In many workings of the German legend of Faust, the protagonist is an alchemist or necromancer employing the dark arts in pursuit of the elixir of eternal youth and ways to transmute base metal into gold. He promises his soul in return for the secret of life. His quest to unravel the mysteries of nature and extend human potential is regarded as tampering with the divine order. It can only end badly.

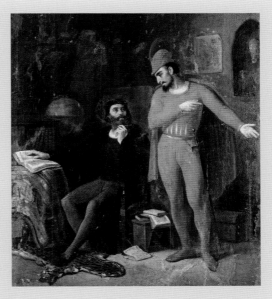

ABOVE: The scholar Faust is tempted by the devil Mephistopheles, and his promise that science will overcome human foibles such as death.

The most famous alchemist was medieval book-dealer and scribe Nicolas Flamel. He worked in Paris in the 14th and 15th centuries, but it took 300 years for his alleged exploits to pass into legend. He reputedly uncovered a Hebrew text on the pilgrimage trail in Spain containing formulae for secret laws that govern the workings of the universe. After deciphering the symbols, together with his wife Perenelle, he formulated the Philosopher's Stone (which turns base metal to gold) and the elixir of life, which through "transmutation of the soul" made the couple immortal. It worked: he lived into his 80s and pops up in most centuries in bestselling books and films, from Victor Hugo's *Notre Dame de Paris* to Dan Brown's *The Da Vinci Code* to the Harry Potter novel named for their invention.

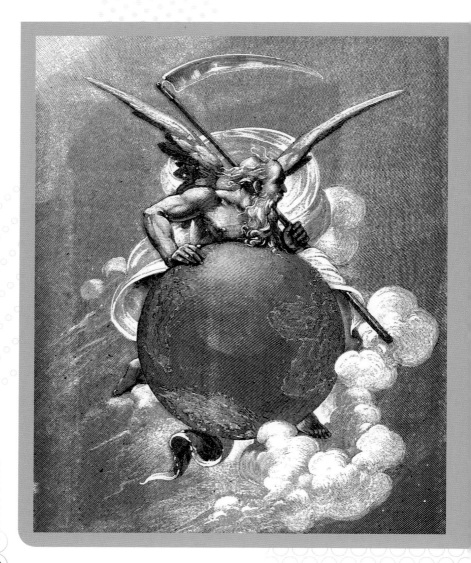

Old father time

Perhaps one of the most benevolent depictions of ageing, along with Father Christmas or the fairy godmother, is the winged figure of Old Father Time, who brings gifts for all, but especially the deserving young. In his earliest incarnations he holds a scythe, suggesting a return from reaping the goodness of nature, and offers the fruits of the earth, nodding to the ever-renewing cycle of the agricultural year. His other gift is a daughter, Truth.

In an earlier incarnation, he is old Chronos, one of two primordial deities present at the beginning of time (*kronos* in Greek). His emblem, too, is a sickle and he is patron of harvest as well as a wielder of formidable forces of destruction. In Roman mythology, Old Father Time is Saturn, his symbol a serpent eating its tail, eternal regeneration. The planet Saturn was considered the planet of old age – the slowest of the planets, steady, dry, serious. Not until after the 11th century does Death wield the sickle and hourglass, connotations of time cut short and running out.

LEFT: In this engraving from 1881, Earth travels through space transported by Old Father Time in benevolent winged form.

Part 1

LONGEVITY BODY:
active, mobile, balanced

What kind of body should we aspire to as we age? One that's agile and mobile, able to do all the things we want it to do, with a balanced skeleton that keeps our frame upright, strong bones to support us securely, supple joints that help us bend and turn, and muscles that contract and extend happily to power us through the day. Then movement is fluid, activity enjoyable and rest comes easily. The muscles and brain remember what we could do when we were younger and life doesn't feel that different.

Sure, there are changes in our muscles, bones and fitness capacity as we age – physically we peak before the age of 35 – but the more active we stay, the more we keep those changes in check. Maximizing physiology keeps our performance as good as it can be as we move through the decades.

So, what happens to us physically from our 30s? Muscle mass and strength decline by 30–50 per cent between the ages of 30 and 80, although it isn't until we reach 60, and especially in our 70s, that dramatic changes in muscle strength, agility, flexibility and endurance kick in. The cardiorespiratory system declines after the age of 40. Aerobic capacity (the amount of oxygen the body uses during peak performance) decreases until we have about 30 per cent less capacity by age 65. Men's performance after 40 declines faster than women's, no matter how much exercise is taken.

The good news is, whatever our age, we can modify the declines in muscle mass and aerobic capacity simply by being more active and doing some resistance training. Everyone knows a sedentary middle-ager who turned life around by training for a marathon or long-distance cycle, and data from Strava app users show that people in their 40s finish marathons an average two minutes quicker than runners in their 20s. Studies show it's possible to up your aerobic capacity by 25 per cent, which, in effect, makes you 20 years younger. In the Dallas Bed Rest and Training Study (see page 44), men in their 50s got back the cardio fitness they had as 20-year-olds. They reversed the effects of 30 years of not exercising in just six months.

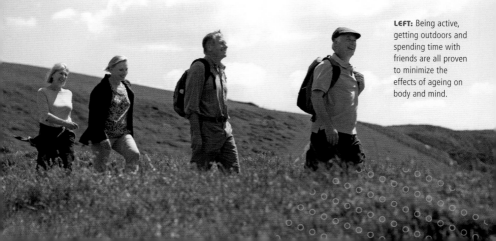

LEFT: Being active, getting outdoors and spending time with friends are all proven to minimize the effects of ageing on body and mind.

A long-lived body is a balanced body, one that holds us upright against gravity and keeps us safe and steady. Falls are the prime reason we lose our ability to stay active and independent as we age – and after 60 the number of falls increases dramatically.

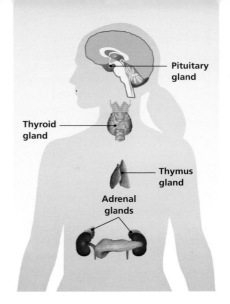

ABOVE: Ageing affects the functioning of the endocrine system and the glands and organs that produce hormones and regulate key body functions.

Rebalance hormones

A balanced body maintains good hormonal balance, too. These chemical messengers have a massive influence on every body system, and as we age, the organs and glands of the endocrine system change. The number of hormones produced, how well they're metabolized and the sensitivity of hormone receptors all change, often declining. Some suggest the effects of ageing are mostly to do with declining hormones – the effects, including increased body fat and decreased muscle mass, are spookily similar to those experienced by young adults with hormone deficiencies.

The pituitary gland, controller of the endocrine system, regulates hormones affecting growth, and with age it gets smaller and less efficient. Loss of growth hormone, which stimulates cell growth, metabolism and muscle development, affects the strength and mass of muscle and bone, plus heart and immune function. Produced in the adrenal gland, Dehydroepiandrosterone (DHEA, aka the youth hormone) protects the cardiovascular, neurological and immune systems, and acts against diabetes and obesity. It declines quickly after age 30. The thyroid gland produces fewer hormones, too, meaning a lower metabolic rate and increasing levels of fat. Cells become less sensitive to insulin secreted from the pancreas post-50, and glucose metabolism slows. Increasing amounts of parathyroid hormone affect calcium levels and contribute to osteoporosis, as does the significant, menopause-triggering loss of oestrogen and progesterone in women. In men, testosterone decreases, but more gradually. Melatonin, which regulates the sleep-wake body clock, also wanes, and that can affect the sleep cycle.

Put simply, declining hormones means decreased leanness and bone mass, increased fat and insulin resistance, reduced immunity and libido, more fatigue and problems regulating body heat, not to mention increased risk of heart disease and depression. Surely to reverse the effects we just replace those declining hormones? That doesn't seem to affect longevity, and the side-effects of hormone supplementing aren't well enough researched, experts suggest.

How do we rebalance the hormonal system then? More exercise! And enough sleep. Exercise seems to help maintain the endocrine system and may help to stabilize hormonal activity over the decades. Thirty minutes of resistance training working the large muscle groups, for example, activates the secretion of hormones, increasing the concentration circulating in the blood; effects persist after a session. Aerobic exercise modifies changes caused by ageing in the way the hypothalamus and pituitary glands work together; triggers the pituitary gland to release more hormones, building bone and muscle; and stimulates the thyroid to regulate body temperature, heart rate

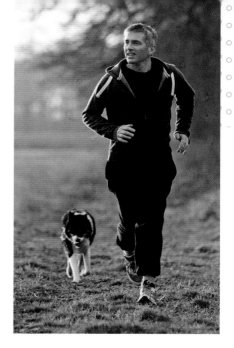

ABOVE: Exercise promotes the release of endorphins, hormones that trigger feelings of positivity and help us want to stay more active.

and blood pressure, while increasing sensitivity to insulin. Exercise also provokes the release of endorphins, the feel-good hormone that wards off the negative effects of stress and makes us feel more motivated to remain active.

Women have most to gain from becoming more active, mobile and balanced with each decade. We tend to become more sedentary with age, and also undergo more dramatic changes in hormone levels, with a greater risk of losing strength, muscle and bone mass ("musculoskeletal atrophy"), making it much harder for the body to function to its full capacity.

All our bodies are programmed to age, but experts find it tricky to tell the difference between physical changes related to age and those resulting from lifestyle. The takeaway message is that we can reset our bodies with exercise. Perhaps more importantly, this helps reset how we perceive the ageing body – not as frail and stiff, but as beautifully resourceful and capable of continual change.

BLESSED SLEEP

Sleep plays a vital rebalancing role. As we sleep, key hormones are released – growth hormone, melatonin, prolactin, insulin – that help repair tissue, regulate immunity and appetite, keep the body clock rhythmic and convert food into energy. People who suffer from insomnia tend to have higher levels of the stress-related hormones linked to short-term memory problems, high blood pressure and increased risk of heart disease.

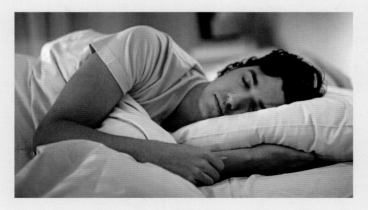

ABOVE: Sleep patterns may shift with age, but requirements for deep sleep remain just the same.

The warrior archetype

It can be useful as we age to rethink the archetypes we keep in our heads. These serve us, consciously or unconsciously, as role models, and if we refresh them every few years they can help us negotiate and refine what it is to be a man or woman in each new phase of life. This helps us make better choices so that we keep fulfilling our potential.

Psychologist Carl Jung pioneered the idea of archetypes and their role in the collective unconscious. He taught that human experience honed over thousands of generations produced thought patterns and instincts common to all of us, wherever we live and in whichever era. These universal archetypes manifest in folk tales and customs, dreams and fantasies, literature and imagery, accounting for similarities in symbols, rituals and stories across diverse cultures and times.

As we age, different aspects of these universal archetypes can come into focus or seem more relevant, and they can be especially helpful in guiding us through times of change. There are male and female archetypes, and regardless of gender, we can identify with aspects of both.

The active male archetype is the warrior, a mature masculine character we learn to grow into. This is someone with distinct goals and clear thinking, strong in limb, secure in posture and steady in focus. He is ever-alert, ready to act but equally able to hold back. He has the courage to tackle what requires his attention, and the intelligence to rein in resources and conserve energy where necessary. There is efficiency in his movements. He is flexible and can move with ease from a poised position of strength and readiness to

"The true art of living in this world is more like a wrestler's than a dancer's skill. That is, to teach a man or woman that whatsoever falls upon them they may be prepared and ready for it, so that nothing may overthrow them or cast them down."

MARCUS AURELIUS

strike a decisive blow to front or back, implementing a decision motivated by principles and discipline. This is a good archetype to keep in mind as the active body ages.

Marcus Aurelius, Emperor of Ancient Rome and perhaps the ultimate warrior-philosopher, wrote of the *dogmata*, the presiding principles and truths we choose to live by. He advised that in times of pressure or distraction we withdraw inside to rest in our *dogmata*, pictured as an inner sanctum of truth that restores and refreshes while promoting strength and security.

The active female stereotype is Diana in the Roman world, Artemis in the Greek pantheon. She is the independent huntress roaming the wilderness with her bow and arrows, ready to protect, rescue or punish. She is steadfast and will survive, an equal of her brother, Apollo. In a recent incarnation she's Katniss, protagonist of the dystopian stories of *The Hunger Games*. She has inspired a fierce and righteous generation of young women, sure of their power and ready to take on authority and fight for justice and freedom, for the

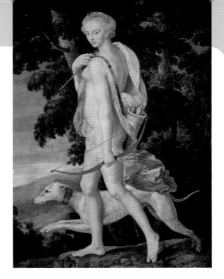

ABOVE: The Roman goddess Diana, the huntress, is ever-young and both a fearless stalker and life-affirming protectoress of women. She leads her female disciples in midnight revels and shameless marauding.

rights of women, children and the natural world. As older women, we too can tap this Generation K energy as we head into the "wilderness" of a world that seems intolerant of the ageing body. Contemplating the Diana archetype can help us remember the energy of the tomboy years and reconnect with the self-confident and unselfconsciously active girls we were before the hormones of puberty kicked in. Connecting to this archetype gives us a way of channelling the eternal energy of youth.

Cultivating warrior energy

This yoga posture, known as Warrior Pose II (*Virabhadrasana II*), helps to cultivate a warrior quality of mind while building strength and balance in the lower body and a focused and flexible upper body.

1. Stand with your feet about 1.2m (4ft) apart and stretch out your arms, extending through to the fingertips – your heels should be beneath your wrists.

2. Turn your right foot inward slightly, and your left foot out by 90 degrees to face the short front end of your mat (if using). Bend your left knee so it's positioned above your left ankle. To keep your knee safe, make sure

it's heading toward your little toe not dropping inward. Press into the outer edge of your right foot and lift from the arch; feel that lift extend up to your inner thigh.

3. Keep your torso anchored over the midline of your body and look down your left arm. Fix your gaze on your middle fingernail and soften your eyes. Hold for a few breaths.

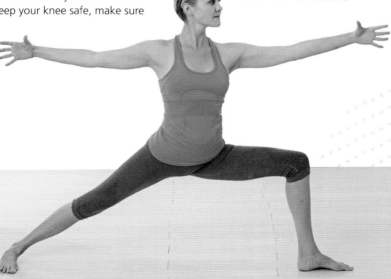

4. Let's move now. Inhale and extend out through your hands. As you exhale, bend your elbows to bring your hands toward each other in front of your chest. As you inhale, extend your arms again, keeping your shoulder blades together. Repeat for ten breaths in and out, visualizing a golden ball of energy at your chest.

Cup your fingers softly to support its energy. As you move, sense the stability and strength in your lower body, and the flexibility and focus in your upper body.

5. Exhale to straighten your front leg and rest with hands on hips before turning your feet to repeat to the right.

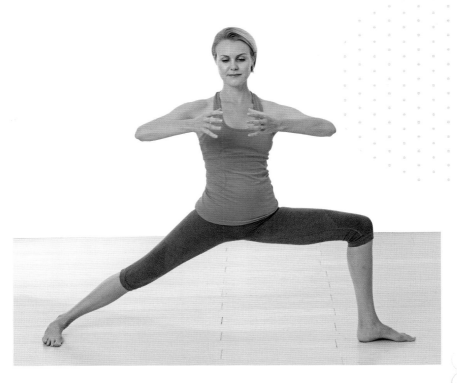

Exercise for a longer life

What's the best way to future-proof your body, whatever your age? Exercise. It's the number-one contributor to longevity, lowering the risk of the conditions most likely to cut life short: heart disease, high blood pressure, some cancers, obesity, Alzheimer's.

The US Office of Disease Prevention and Health Promotion says regular exercise seems to reduce mortality by more than a quarter and increase life expectancy by more than two years (over a sedentary life). Put bluntly, the less activity we do as we age, the more likely we are to die.

BENEFITS OF EXERCISE AS WE AGE

- Lowered risk of heart disease and high blood pressure, diabetes, cancer, osteoporosis, obesity, Alzheimer's and dementia
- Stronger bones and muscles, better balance
- Improved immunity
- More efficient digestion, metabolism and waste elimination
- Decreased mortality

Keep moving

Whatever your age and preferred form of exercise, the most important thing you can do for your health is to move more. Mobility is the key to better posture, stronger bones, more powerful muscles and increased agility. Continue moving and you maximize your chances of preserving a high quality of life and independence into old age, not to mention reducing the risk of chronic disease and injury and improving your mood.

Many of the physiological signs we associate with ageing – weaker muscles, loss of strength and endurance, stiff joints, increased fat – are simply a result of inactivity. A sedentary life is associated with increased falls, depression, blood clots and swelling. In fact, it's tricky, say the experts, to distinguish between *real* age-related decline and changes caused by an inactive lifestyle. As we get older, reduced mobility is a risk factor for some nasty words, such as morbidity, hospitalization, disability, mortality.

The good news is that even if you're inactive now, once you start to exercise

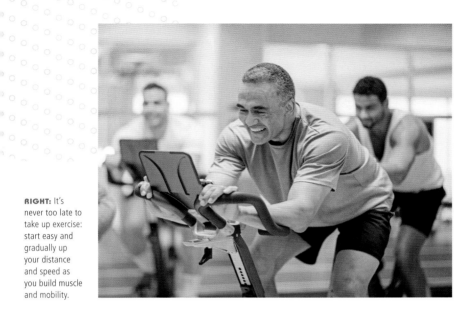

RIGHT: It's never too late to take up exercise: start easy and gradually up your distance and speed as you build muscle and mobility.

you begin to restore function and improve both life expectancy and the quality of those extended years. Even the frailest of us. A study in the *New England Journal of Medicine* found that nursing-home residents showed an average 97 per cent increase in strength after just ten weeks of resistance training. The Harvard Alumni Health Study found that previously sedentary men who began exercising after the age of 45 had a 24 per cent lower rate of death than their sedentary peers.

In order to maintain mobility, it's useful to prioritize key areas of the body – strengthening the lower limbs and core support (see pages 78–97), maintaining lateral movement in the sides of the body (see pages 116–23), and looking after the lower back (see pages 124–31). Warming up well and active recovery become more important with age, and as the decades pass we may find we're working as much on maintaining form and rehabilitation after an injury as on building new skills. But it's important to keep pushing at the edges when we feel comfortable in an activity – applying a little "healthy" stress by trying something new, or doing something for a short while longer or a little harder than usual, strengthens the body's tissues and keeps them healthy.

In 1966 five 20-year-old men went to bed for three weeks, monitored by researchers at the University of Texas Southwestern Medical School. Their bodies underwent a drastic ageing process. In just three weeks their heart rate, blood pressure, muscle strength and body fat went from healthy to the equivalent of men twice their age. The Dallas Bed Rest and Training Study team then put them on an eight-week exercise regime. This didn't just reverse the damage, it left them healthier than when they'd started the trial.

The five men re-engaged with the programme 30 years later. Now in their 50s, all had worse cardiac health and increased body fat, but still weren't as debilitated as after three weeks of bed rest back in their 20s. The five started a six-month graded programme of steady aerobic exercise (walking, jogging, cycling). Amazingly, it reset their heart rate, blood pressure and aerobic output at their 20-year-old levels. With exercise alone they wound back the clock 30 years.

Be balanced

A strong balance – or vestibular – system is important in keeping us active and able to engage effectively in exercise. The system uses a network of peripheral sensory organs and neurons to process sensory input in order to tell us where we are in space, how fast and in which direction we're travelling, and where our head is in relation to gravity.

As children, we move freely in all directions for hours at a time, and this develops a strong vestibular system. Once our movements become more restricted, as they inevitably do while we settle into a smaller range of habitual patterns through school and work, the balance system stops working as well as it could. When our muscles lose power with age, our flexibility and range of movement in the joints decline, and the body compensates for injury by adapting its movements – this is when balance really suffers. Dizziness and falls follow. Non-specific dizziness is the health issue most frequently reported to doctors by older people, and is connected not only with increased falls, but with depression, fear, social isolation and an overall reduction in function. Sadly, fall-related injuries are one of the top leading causes of death in elderly people.

To counter this decline we should act more like children, chucking ourselves in all directions all the time. Instead of being upright for hours we need to go

> "And is not the body spoiled by rest
> and idleness, but preserved for a
> long time by motion and exercise?"
>
> **PLATO**

upside down, stand on one leg, hop, use a balance board, balance on our hands, hang from bars. This builds core strength while sharpening our balance and sensory systems. Movement in diverse directions (even leaning is good) "perturbs" our centre of gravity, which teaches the body ways to respond to bring us back into balance. If you're a fidgeter, you might find it brings better focus, too. Yoga and martial arts are incredibly useful in developing the vestibular and sensory systems.

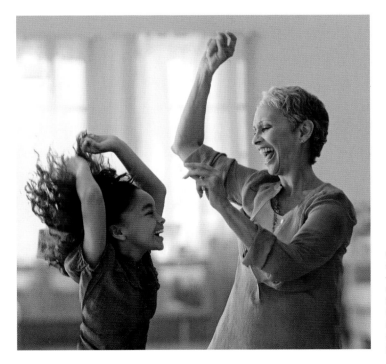

LEFT: Act like a child more often – ideally with a child, to gain the considerable benefits (to all ages) of connecting the generations.

LONGEVITY BODY

45

Maintain muscle

We reach peak muscle mass between the ages of 20 and 30. Over the following two decades we slowly lose muscle mass and, with it, strength. From the age of 50 more than 15 per cent of our strength fades per decade as the number of muscle fibres, nerves and neurons declines, and between the ages of 20 and 75 we lose more than half of our "fast-twitch" muscle fibres, meaning it takes us longer to respond to stimuli. The loss is connected with reducing levels of growth hormone and testosterone alongside a reduction in our ability to process protein.

CHECK YOUR WAIST

The composition of the body changes with age, so we have less muscle and more fat. Hormonal changes mean fat tends to congregate around the abdomen. Keep a watch on your waist. As it gets bigger, so do the risks of heart disease and stroke, type-2 diabetes and some cancers. Here's when you should try and lose weight:

- **Women:** waist measures more than 80cm (31.5in); risk increases substantially over 88cm (34.5in).

- **Men:** waist measures more than 94cm (37in); risk increases substantially over 102cm (40in) or 90cm (35in) for Asian men.

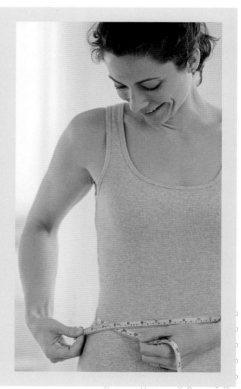

RIGHT: Regardless of your BMI, height or weight, waist measurement is a good indicator of your risk from key diseases associated with ageing.

The decline speeds up rapidly after 60 and any time we're sedentary – studies suggest that older muscle may be more sensitive to short periods of inactivity than younger people's muscle. As we lose muscle, so endurance and power in the lower limbs reduces and our ability to keep up a series of repetitive movements declines. Less massy muscle means slower reaction times and coordination, increased risk of fatigue and injury and slower muscle repair. The body starts to compensate to keep us upright, which can lead to postural problems. For instance, many of us adjust the angle of the spine to keep our bodyweight in balance, which can lead to curvature of the spine, and the extra weight imposed through the hip and knee joints puts undue stress on them. Resistance training (lifting, pulling or pushing against an opposing force) is the best way to maintain muscle mass and strength.

If you go to a gym, ask a trainer who works with older people to set a strength-training programme to suit your age, fitness level and gender and ensure the right blend of high-intensity to stability work, so you build muscle efficiently and safely. A trainer will also advise on how to mix in aerobic exercise.

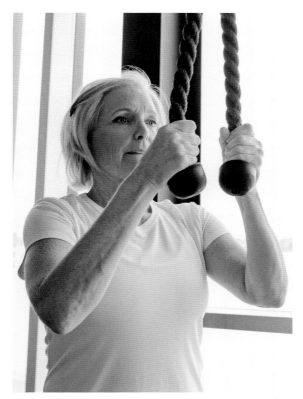

LEFT: Strength-training the upper body also supports the muscles we use for breathing, which weaken with age.

Build bone

Bone density peaks in our late 20s, and declines by around 0.5 per cent per year after the age of 40. The mineral content of bones lessens, making them more fragile and brittle, and micro-cracks increase with age, reducing toughness. Frail bones affect around a quarter of people over 60, leading to increased risk of fracture. As the skeleton weakens it becomes less able to support the load of the body (and to serve as a calcium reservoir), leading to changes in posture, gait and balance and a reduced range of movement, all increasing the risk of falls. Some bones are particularly susceptible to structural change and damage, including the hips and the tibia and femur in the legs.

Joints are affected by a decline in cartilage, the cushioning between bones. As this thins, joints become more prone to injury and susceptible to the effects of stress. Increased rigidity in older ligaments and tendons also contributes to stiffness and a reduction in range of movement in the joints.

Osteoporosis is not a condition of ageing *per se*, but since it's associated with loss of bone mass and strength it's seen more often in older than younger people. It leaves the bones fragile and prone to increased risk of fracture, and makes the joints vulnerable, particularly the hips and wrists. A light, thin frame is a risk factor, as is a reduced level of

oestrogen from menopause onward – but men are also subject to a decrease in bone mineral density, especially smokers.

Weight-bearing resistance training is the best way to preserve bone density – studies show increased bone mass in the legs and backs of older people who work out with weights, while regular walkers build bone in the hips and lower back. Exercise that incorporates balance skills is useful to ward off falls, while moving through a range of movements and varying forms of exercise protects the joints from overwork.

Preserve flexibility

It's not just muscles and bones that are affected by age. The matrix of collagen-rich soft tissue that connects them plays a key role in how well we are able to maintain a healthy range of movement over the decades. Ligaments – tissue connecting bone to bone – reduce in elasticity with age, restricting movement in the joints. Tendons – which attach muscle to bone – stiffen as their water content decreases with age. This makes them more likely to tear (and take longer to heal), making us less flexible and less stable.

Bodywork and movement therapists often focus on the web of connective tissue, or fascia, enveloping our muscles, bones and organs. Its weave of collagen fibres glued together by water-absorbent mucus keeps everything connected,

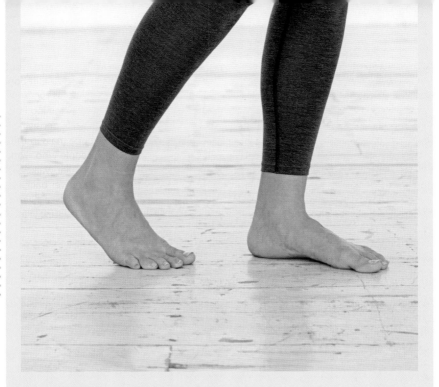

ABOVE: Keep the feet and ankles supple and responsive and it's easier to stay active and maintain a good range of movement through the body.

LOOK TO THE FEET

The building of balance and good gait starts in the feet and legs. A 2011 Australian clinical trial found a combination of feet exercises, shoe inserts and advice on footwear reduced falls by 36 per cent a year. Grounding exercises for the lower body based on yoga and tai chi (see page 79) can help us find the combination of strength and relaxation we need to stay upright and agile.

supportively bound together, yet able to slide over each other smoothly when required. Imagine a web of netting running sleekly around every organ, muscle and bone, like a mesh bag around onions – tightness or disruption in one area causes compression or disconnection elsewhere in the net, and this affects the movement and stability of the whole.

Author Tom Myers developed a way of mapping the fascia connections running up and down and around the body (like the meridians in Traditional Chinese Medicine). One of these "anatomy trains" runs up the back of the body – starting at the toes, it heads down the sole of the foot and up the backs of the legs, then moves up the back and over the top of the head. Tightness in the backs of the calves, for example, can lead to disruption further up the train, maybe causing restriction in the shoulders or neck.

Fascia loses elasticity after our 50s. Injury and habit as well as loss of hydration in the glue that allows tissue to stretch and glide results in tightness that prevents the body from working as a whole and interrupts our natural range of movement. Sitting is particularly disruptive – the amount of time we spend seated is increasing in every age group and has been named an "independent risk factor for health" by Harvard's Sightlines longevity project.

To keep the fascia supple and to build its resilience and elasticity, try yoga, tai chi or qigong. Whole-body movements are recommended over the kind of spot-focused repetitive actions provided by a weights machine or formula fitness class (though these are good for aerobic and endurance training, see page 55). The most effective exercise for keeping the fascia supple replicates everyday movements, building in the surprise and variation you don't get from practising sets of reps over and over to a count.

Other movement therapies based on structural integration, such as the Feldenkrais Method, are effective at promoting natural function throughout the frame, easing out injury and preventing small twinges leading to more debilitating problems.

THE FELDENKRAIS METHOD

This teaches how to read feedback from the senses and use it to refine movement and undo unhelpful patterns caused by habit or injury, thereby improving mobility and building balance and dexterity. To tune in like this increases sensitivity and helps us find more comfortable and natural ways of moving. Notice how your body feels when you're not on automatic!

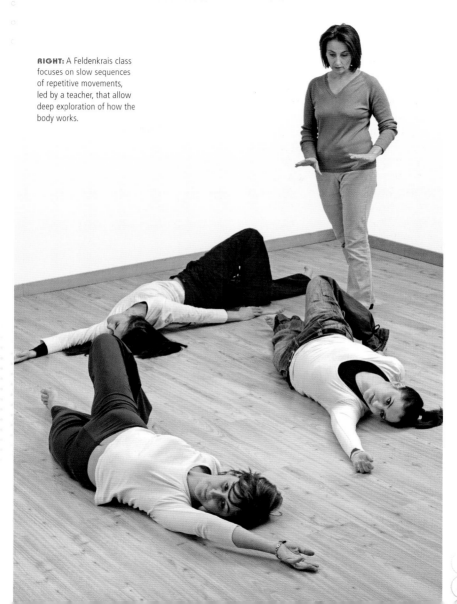

RIGHT: A Feldenkrais class focuses on slow sequences of repetitive movements, led by a teacher, that allow deep exploration of how the body works.

Tune in to your moving body

Adapted from the Feldenkrais Method, this exercise builds awareness of where your body feels at ease and where movement is more effortful.

1. Start by lying on your back, knees bent and feet flat on the floor, hip-width apart. Extend your arms to the side. Notice where the breath is in your body and how your pelvis, shoulders and head feel against the floor and in relation to each other. Spend some time on this.

2. Roll onto one side so your hips, knees, shoulders and arms are stacked on top of each other, palms together. Look toward your palms with the side of your head supported by the floor (or a folded blanket if that's more comfortable).

3. Slowly slide your top hand forward onto the floor, then back over the palm onto your lower arm. Repeat a few times. Notice how your knees move and how this affects your head, which might roll.

4. Very gently glide your top arm forward, then up around your head in an arc. If your fingertips reach the floor allow them to drag. Let your head follow the movement. Now let your lower arm follow the arc around your head, and your knees roll so eventually you're facing the other direction, with palms, knees and hips stacked.

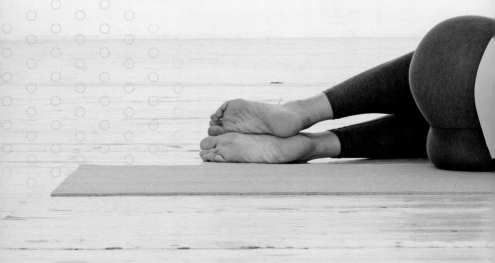

5. Repeat to the other side. Slide your top arm forward and back, then glide it up and around your head, again allowing your lower arm and hips to follow in a smooth, soft, rolling movement. Notice any areas that feel stiff and move more slowly around them. Consider which parts of your body contribute to the action and which hinder it. How could you ease the movement? Repeat four or five times in each direction, focusing on the quality of your movement.

6. Finish on your back again, knees bent and feet hip-width apart, arms easy by your sides. Notice your breathing – does it feel easier or deeper? Has the way your pelvis and shoulders and head rest on the floor changed? Observe your body before rolling to one side and pushing up to a seated position.

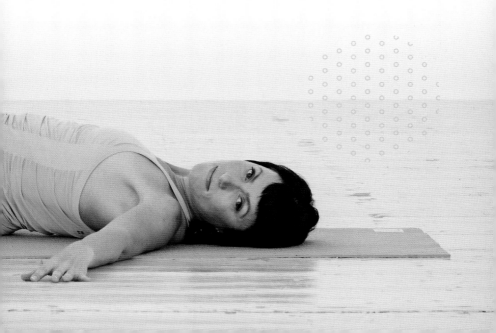

Activities to future-proof your body

Exercise reduces our biological age. People who are active live longer and retain physical function for longer, but studies show that the older we get, the less likely we are to do the three 30-minute sessions of moderate-intensity exercise recommended each week, and figures are worse for women than men.

The effects of a sedentary life are as great in terms of losses in functional capacity as the effects of ageing. By exercising we roll back the years. Which kind of exercise is best? Different studies find that cycling, high-intensity interval training (HIIT) and running offer impressive benefits in maximizing health as we age. Yoga and tai chi rate impressively well, too.

THE ESSENTIALS

As we age we need the same amount of exercise as younger adults. To improve the health of the heart and lungs, muscle strength and bone density, a combination of cardio workouts, weight training and stretching is recommended, as follows:

Weekly longevity formula

- **Aerobic and endurance training:** at least 150 minutes of moderate-intensity activity (30 minutes x 5) or 75 minutes of vigorous activity, or a combination of the two.
- **Strength and resistance training:** two or more sessions working the large muscles in the legs, hips, back, abdomen, chest, shoulders and arms.
- **Flexibility and balance training:** use as a warm-up and cool-down in each exercise session to promote body awareness and coordination and reduce the risk of injury.

NEW TO EXERCISE

If you're frail or new to exercise, build up to your 150 minutes of weekly aerobic exercise with ten-minute mini-sessions. Start slowly with moderate-intensity activities, such as walking or cycling over flat ground, and build in intensity over several weeks as your stamina develops. If you feel dizzy, get cramp or feel pain in your joints or chest, shoulders or arms, slow down and stop exercising.

If you have a health condition, talk to your doctor about which activities would best suit you before you start to exercise.

EXERCISING SAFELY

• Warm up for five to ten minutes, gradually increasing your pace and the size of your movements.

• Cool down for five to ten minutes after exercising, by slowing down as gradually as you warmed up, then stretch out the large muscles in your legs and arms.

• Vary the exercise you do to avoid the risk of stress to joints or muscles.

• If running, make sure to vary the terrain, running in the park and on the track as well as unforgiving pavements.

• Good form is more important than number of reps, distance covered or vinyasas (flowing sequences of yoga poses) completed. When you notice your posture or breathing slipping or your jaw clenching, slow down and become more mindful of your movement.

Aerobic and endurance training

Any activity that gets the large muscles moving rhythmically for a sustained period of time and increases the pulse and breathing rate is good aerobic training – such as cycling, walking, running, swimming and racquet sports. These develop the body's ability to deliver oxygen and nutrients around the body and remove waste, and after a few weeks increase endurance. This is the best way to improve cardiovascular function (lowering the resting heart rate and blood pressure) and may help counter bone-density loss in postmenopausal women. It makes us more sensitive to insulin (reducing risk of diabetes), boosts good cholesterol and enhances mood, sleep and memory.

Training three times a week improves your functional capacity. The more you keep it up (over 20 weeks), the better the improvements will be.

Aim for a moderate-intensity workout, so you feel warm and out of breath but can keep up a conversation. Add in vigorous activity where you can, so you get hot and can't really talk. Short sharp bursts of activity bring extra benefits for heart health and lead to faster recovery times.

Good choice – cycling

Cycling 30 miles (48km) per week lowers your risk of premature death by 41 per cent, according to the findings of a large five-year study by the University of Glasgow. That's 6 miles (9.8km) per day five days a week – maybe the distance you travel to work? The study suggested that commuting by bike reduces the risk of developing cardiovascular disease by 46 per cent and cancer by 45 per cent.

Cycling was found to be more effective than walking – probably because of

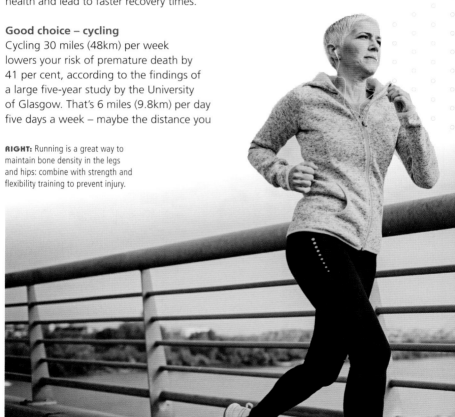

RIGHT: Running is a great way to maintain bone density in the legs and hips: combine with strength and flexibility training to prevent injury.

the longer distances covered and the intensity involved in navigating hills and sprinting away at junctions. Another study conducted by King's College London found that cyclists aged 55–79 were physically younger than their peers.

Lots of us worry about the risks to health of air pollution when we cycle, and fear of road-traffic accidents seems to be a big factor in deterring people from getting on their bikes. But statistics show that the diseases associated with ageing – heart disease, stroke, obesity – are much

more of a risk to our health than cycling accidents. And although cycling in traffic-filled urban environments *does* expose us to pollutants such as nitrogen dioxide and carbon monoxide, epidemiological research from Cambridge University suggests that the health benefits of cycling far outweigh the dangers of pollution. For instance, you'd need to cycle in London for just under 10 hours for the pollutant harm to outweigh the benefits of physical activity. Unless you are a cycle courier in Delhi, the WHO's most-polluted city, urban cycling is much more health-giving than not cycling at all.

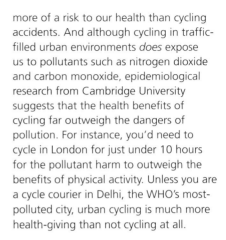

Good choice – running

In one data-analysis study, running was found to be the single most effective exercise to extend life. It suggested that runners tend to live three years longer than those who don't run – even if they smoke, drink, are overweight or have high blood pressure – and have a 25–40 per cent reduced risk of dying prematurely. Slow running was effective, and even five minutes made a difference.

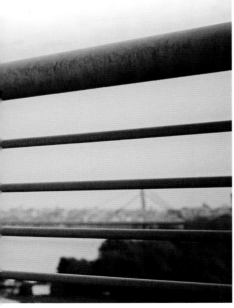

TIP: One hour's running reportedly adds seven hours extra life, though these gains plateau after approximately four hours of running each week. The increase in life length gained by running is capped at around three years.

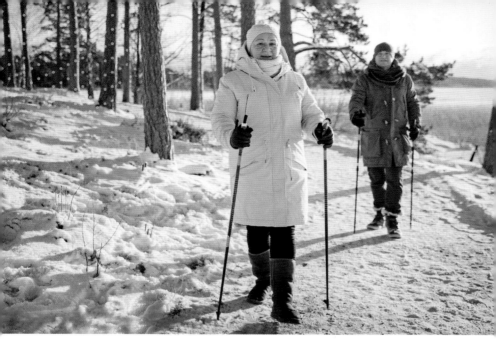

Good choice – brisk walking

The most accessible and perhaps the safest way to start exercising is by walking – and just 25 minutes of brisk walking each day can add up to seven years to life span. In a large, long-term study, moderate-intensity walking brought about similar reductions in risk for high blood pressure as vigorous running – and the more of it you can do each week, the greater the benefits. Walking helps to maintain bone density and cognitive function and eases depression, and covering 2.5–3km (1½–2 miles) a week at a brisk pace also reduces the risk of cardiovascular disease.

ABOVE: Nordic walking exercises the arms and upper body and encourages good posture, while getting us out into nature.

RIGHT: Take the Plank challenge to activate all the muscles of the front of the body – the ones we switch off while sitting.

TIP: One minute's vigorous activity has the same benefits as two minutes' moderate activity.

HIGH-INTENSITY INTERVAL TRAINING (HIIT)

The idea of fitting brief bursts of very vigorous activity into moderate aerobic activity seems particularly effective for older people. Such a regime may also be kinder to an ageing body than more drawn-out periods of moderate activity, which can be draining, tough on the joints and take time to recover from.

Spinning or interval-training classes, hill riding and Ashtanga Yoga are all options. In studies, HIIT had most impact on endurance, with even a short time making a difference. In one study conducted by the Mayo Clinic, older people seemed to have a more intense reaction to HIIT than younger people, and it corrected declines in the mitochondria (see page 15) associated with ageing. HIIT activated 400 genes in ageing muscle cells compared with 170 in moderate exercisers and 74 in weightlifters. In this study people trained three times a week on exercise bikes (four minutes hard pedalling followed by a three-minute rest, repeated four times in total).

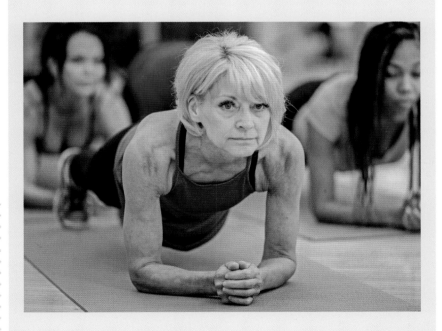

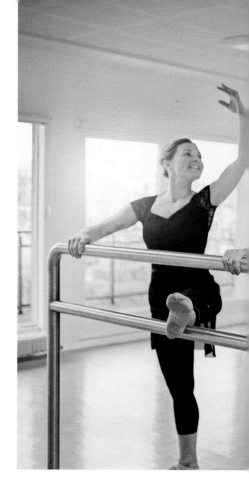

RIGHT: It's never too late to begin ballet or rekindle a childhood fantasy. Look for teachers trained to work with adult learners.

Strength and resistance training

Exercise that gets the muscles working repetitively against a force or weight is the best way to minimize age-related muscle deterioration, protect bone density and build strength in the tendons and ligaments. Activities such as climbing stairs, squats, press-ups, sit-ups and weight workouts help with balance, regulate blood pressure and blood-sugar levels and seem to stimulate a rise in growth hormone and sensitivity to insulin.

You can start training at any age and increase your muscle tissue (and strength and power) substantially – studies of people over 70 have shown a doubling of muscle strength in ten weeks.

Use free weights, machine weights or your own body weight and start with 8–12 repetitions of an exercise, increasing the weight or number of repetitions as your strength grows. If you do strength training every day, alternate the muscles you work to give them a rest day.

Good choice – exercise in water

Water resistance works muscles effectively while its buoyancy supports the joints and bodyweight, making this a safe medium if you're recovering from injury or are carrying more weight than is comfortable.

Good choice – dance

Ballet is a good way of building strength in the lower body. In a study at Sydney University, participation in dance reduced falls by 37 per cent, perhaps as a result of increased strength in the lower limbs,

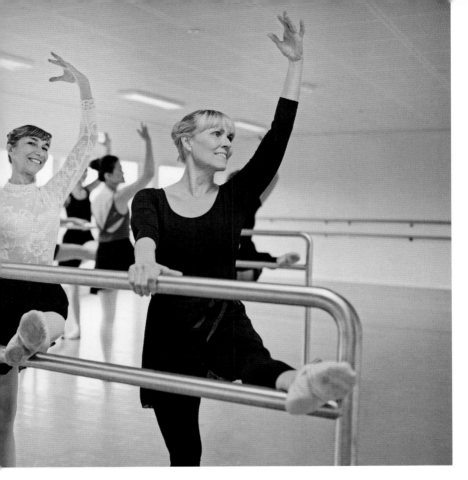

joints and core muscles, alongside increased balance, flexibility and spatial awareness. The small, precise movements in the feet, legs and hips cause less stress than high-impact training, while learning to align the joints – head over shoulders, over hips, over knees – builds good form for all types of weight-training. A barre class builds strength evenly as you switch sides to repeat exercises, leading with both left and right limbs.

Flexibility and balance training

Stretching and posture-awareness exercises help maintain and increase the body's range of motion. By working on the fascia they also play a role in shape-shifting the body. These forms of exercise, such as yoga, tai chi and qigong, also promote balance – falls are reportedly the largest preventable cause of death and injury in the over-65s. Memorizing stretching sequences and switching on the mind-body focus required to self-correct as you practise promotes mental agility and the power to do two things at once.

Stretch the shoulders and upper arms, calves and thighs to warm up before exercising and as a cool-down afterward. This enables you to use muscles more efficiently and effectively as you train and reduces the risk of injury.

Good choice – tai chi and qigong

The slow and continuous low-intensity movements of the martial art tai chi and the traditional Chinese wellness practice qigong are known for their efficacy in preventing and treating the symptoms of many conditions associated with ageing, from arthritic pain to high blood pressure. They offer a brilliant way of rehabilitating the body after injury, especially if you're wary of exercise exacerbating pain.

The smooth meditative movements of the form, the softness of the muscles

and lack of extension in the joints seem helpful for connective tissue. Shifting the bodyweight through a range of positions triggers receptors in the muscles and ligaments to keep the body balanced, which has been shown to help reduce fear of falling. Studies suggest that although tai chi and qigong don't involve weight-bearing or resistance training, they increase bone formation, especially in postmenopausal women. The "held" limb

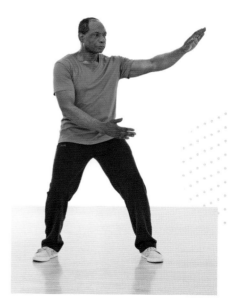

ABOVE: Qigong is the ultimate exercise for people who enjoy balancing energy within the body and the world around them.

and posture positions also seem to build muscular strength in the upper and lower body and core.

Good choice – yoga

Perhaps the most obvious benefits of practising yoga asanas, or postures, are increased flexibility and better balance, coordination and body-awareness. The practice of yoga realigns the posture and gait and frees up areas of stiffness while expanding the range of movement. The focus on breathing and mindful movement has been shown to be helpful for many conditions associated with ageing, including heart disease and high blood pressure, and the relaxation techniques can ease the chronic pain of arthritis and lower back problems, and reduce the medication required to control certain conditions including type-2 diabetes. Yoga is also associated with reducing depression, stress and insomnia and developing mental clarity and concentration.

Yoga builds muscle strength and tone, strengthens the ankles and knees, rehabilitates cartilage in the joints and increases bone density. It shares some of the benefits of aerobic and endurance training, such as lowering the resting heart rate and improving lung function and oxygen take-up during exercise. It also seems to lower blood sugar and bad cholesterol.

STRETCH YOURSELF YOUNGER

A flexible and toned body acts young but might it be biologically younger, too? A 2017 study suggested that yoga can significantly reduce the rate of cellular ageing in healthy people. It looked at the main markers for cellular ageing – DNA damage, oxidative stress, telomere length attrition – which seemed to stabilize after a 12-week yoga and meditation course.

An Indian study found that an intensive 12-week daily yoga practice including Sun Salutations (see page 64) significantly increased levels of growth hormone and DHEA (the so-called youth hormone, see page 35) in people aged 35–55, both of which are linked with longevity. The authors suggested that the Sun Salutations sequence works on the pituitary and adrenal glands, and hypothesized that the mind–body nature of the exercises was key to their efficacy.

Easy sun salutation

This complete yoga practice is an integral part of most yoga traditions. It offers the body a complete workout – forward and back bends, hip openers and digestive stimulants, poses that reverse the effects of gravity, promote circulation and act on the nervous system – while bringing mindful awareness of the breath as you move.

1. Stand with feet together or hip-width apart, palms pressing together at your chest. Feel your weight balanced equally between the front, back and sides of both feet. Feel the stability of your feet, legs and hips and your spine rising out of your pelvis, lifting your upper body.

2. As you take a breath in, reach your arms overhead, looking up if that's comfortable. Feel the lift in the sides of your waist and your chest.

3. Breathing out, fold forward from the hips and place your hands on the floor. Bend your knees if you can't easily straighten your legs. Release your head and neck toward your legs.

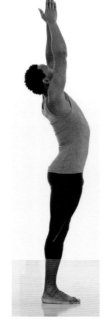

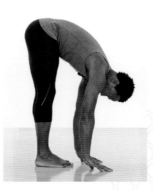

4. Breathing in, raise your chest and head, and step your right leg back into a lunge. Feel a lovely stretch in your lengthened back leg and look forward.

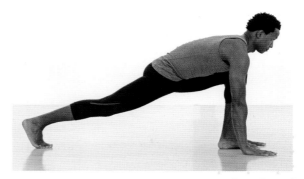

5. As you exhale, step your left leg back in line with your right leg, feet hip-width apart, and drop your head. Push into your hands to guide your chest toward your legs, bending your knees if you need to. This is Downward-facing Dog Pose (*Adhomukha Svanasana*).

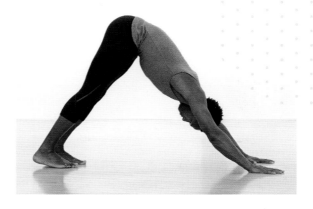

6. On an inhalation, lower both knees to the floor. Then, exhaling, drop your hips back onto your heels, feet together, knees apart. Your chest comes between your knees, arms outstretched without straining, forehead on the floor. Rest here in Child's Pose (*Balasana*) for a full breath (an inhalation and an exhalation).

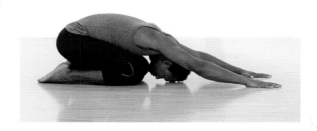

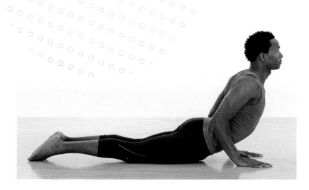

7. Look forward and sweep your chest through between your hands. Inhaling, push up into Cobra Pose (*Bhujangasana*). Stay low in Baby Cobra if your back isn't used to this, just lifting your chest as far as you can with your hands. This strengthens your back muscles.

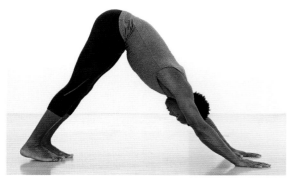

8. On an exhale, push into your hands and raise your hips back to Downward-facing Dog, keeping your knees bent if necessary. Hold for three slow breaths in and out. Push your hips to the ceiling and flatten your hands to the floor, pressing into the base of the thumbs and index fingers.

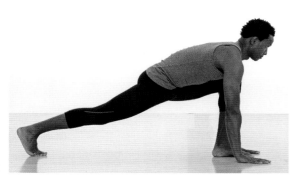

9. As you inhale, look forward and step your left foot between your hands (you may need to hop or pull your foot the last few inches) to come back to a lunge. Feel a lovely stretch on your back leg.

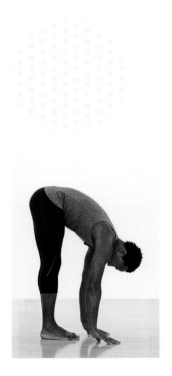
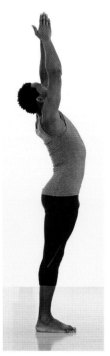
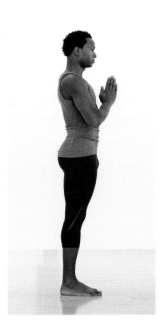

10. Bring your right foot to meet your left foot; then, exhaling, fold forward to bring your chest and head toward your legs (bend your knees if you need to).

11. On an inhale, contract your core muscles and sweep your arms overhead as you straighten up (bend your knees if your back needs more support).

12. Exhale as you lower your arms, bringing your palms together at your chest. Pause. When you feel ready, inhale and sweep your arms overhead to repeat the sequence on the other side of the body, this time stepping back and forward with your right leg. Work up to three or four rounds on each side.

Workout breathing

To fuel your body to keep going during periods of exertion, it's useful to learn how to regulate the breath, elongating the inhalations and exhalations. The type of breathing – *Ujjayi* – used in many of the more fast-flowing forms of yoga can ease the strenuousness of activity and help you tap into reserves of energy. Translating as "victorious" breath, it helps you to the finish line. It's also said to lower raised blood pressure. Learn the technique seated, then once it feels comfortable, apply when powering through yoga sequences, ascending hills or nearing the end of a set of reps.

- To learn the technique, start by watching your regular flow of breath in and out. Then breathe in through your nose for a count of four. Open your mouth slightly and breathe out for a count of four, narrowing your throat and "huffing" the breath out as if misting up a mirror. When you get it right, you'll hear a continuous sound like the sea rushing in and pulling out on a rocky beach.

- To practise *Ujjayi* breath proper, breathe in through your nose, and repeat the sounded out-breath, this time with your mouth closed. It can help to imagine breathing out through a hole in the front of your neck. Keep the throat toned so that you hear the sibilant noise on both the in- and out-breaths, and try to balance the length of the inhalation and exhalation.

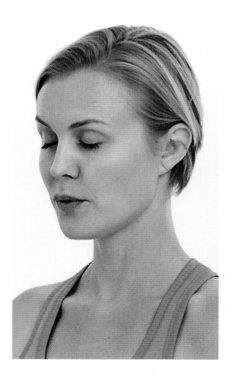

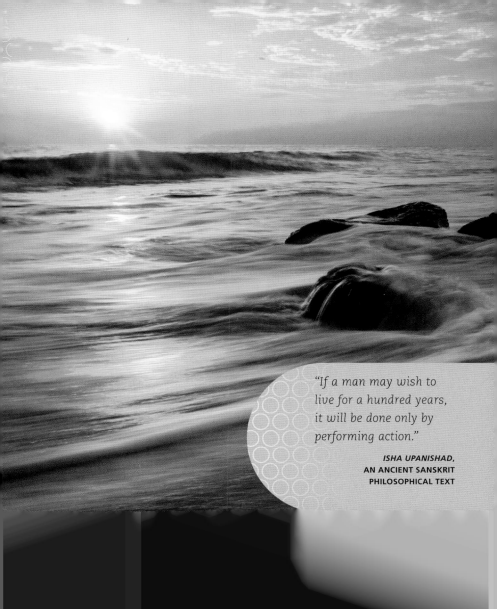

"If a man may wish to live for a hundred years, it will be done only by performing action."

ISHA UPANISHAD,
**AN ANCIENT SANSKRIT
PHILOSOPHICAL TEXT**

Protect your posture

Good movement starts with good posture. If the joints are stacked on top of each other when you are standing and sitting, with a line running through shoulders, hips, knees and ankles, the body's bones will be correctly aligned, including the vertebrae of the spine.

When the bones are aligned, the ligaments that keep the joints in place are unstressed and the muscles work efficiently, making movement less effortful and injury, muscle strain, abnormal wear-and-tear of the joints – and pain – less likely.

Good posture creates space around the ribcage and diaphragm, making it easier to breathe deeply, and by preserving the spine's natural curves around the lower and mid-spine and neck, it prevents back and neck pain. Levelling the hips and shoulders releases stiffness and pain in these vital joints.

A study of the posture of women over 60 identified common postural changes that contribute to stooping and a hunch, including asymmetric shoulder blades, an excessive outward curve in the upper and middle spine and an excessive inward curve in the lower back. Time spent with the

centre of gravity and head shifted forward leads to increased problems with stability, increasing the likelihood of falls as well as pain and degeneration in the hip joints.

If you ask actors to depict an older character, they will stoop, collapse the chest and hamper movement by walking with knees bent. Doing the opposite – adopting a youthful posture with head held high and chest expanded – makes us look younger and feel younger, and makes us more relaxed, confident and focused. The act of widening across the chest and releasing the ribcage has been shown to be mood-enhancing. In studies, it worked particularly well for men, making them feel more dominant and successful and so better able to problem-solve. Adopting a "power pose" – one in which you look confident – increases levels of testosterone and reduces levels of the stress hormone cortisol.

THE PSOAS

One of the most under-sung of the body's muscles, perhaps because it's so hard to feel or visualize, the psoas is vital to our posture, balance and ability to relax effectively. It connects the femur bones at the tops of the legs to the lower back, passing up the front of the pelvis and wrapping around the hips deep inside to attach to the sides of the lumbar vertebrae.

The psoas stabilizes the spine and is critical to our continuing ability to walk and move around effectively, but it decreases in volume as we age – at its healthiest when we are in our 20s, after our 60s it declines dramatically, contributing to problems with the back and gait.

The psoas muscles are contracted except when we lie down, but become tighter and shorten if we spend long periods sitting. To relax and release the psoas for a more natural lumbar curve and freedom of movement, try the Find Your Centre exercise

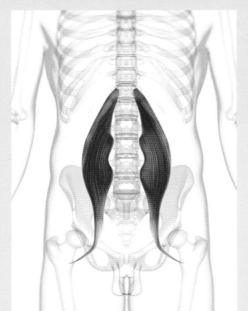

(see page 92), then relax for ten minutes with your calves elevated on the seat of a chair, consciously releasing tension around the pelvis and hips. To stretch the psoas, encouraging the spine to lift, practise Mountain Pose (see page 74).

LEFT: One of the most tricky muscles to access, the psoas lies deep inside our core and responds well to yoga and other "somatic" movement therapies.

Sitting well

Posture matters, especially when we sit, because as we age we tend to sit more often and for longer. The following adjustments help improve your sitting posture, but it's as important to get up every 45 minutes and spend 15 minutes in movement.

1. At a desk or table, sit fully on the seat, backs of your thighs supported and back of the pelvis touching the back of the chair. Lower or raise the seat (or use a footrest, yoga blocks or books) so your feet are flat on the floor, hip-width apart, and positioned beneath your knees, with knees pointing forward. There should be a 90-degree bend at your hips and knees. Make sure the chair back supports your upper back, and there is a nice curve in your lower spine, middle back and the back of your neck. Sit back so that your ears are over your shoulders, which are over your hips. Roll your shoulders up, back and down to check they are even.

2. Imagine there is a balloon fixed to the crown of your head, pulling you up from the back of the neck. Imagine another balloon string lifting your chest from the breastbone, which in turn lifts your chin slightly.

• For computer work, position your screen so your lower arms are parallel to the ground and look straight ahead. You may need an external monitor if you use a laptop; try positioning it on books to raise it to the right height. Visualize your stomach muscles pulling back toward your spine to support your upper body. Core strength is essential for good posture. If this is new to you, don't do more than ten minutes at a sitting.

TIP: Sit on an exercise ball to watch TV – the involuntary micro-movements needed to maintain balance exercise the core muscles that keep us upright and the muscles that stabilize the spine.

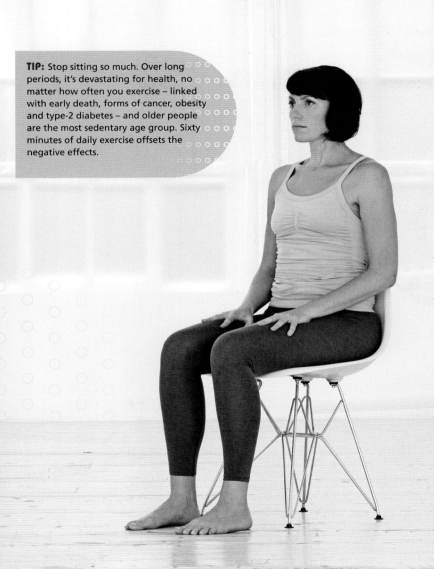

TIP: Stop sitting so much. Over long periods, it's devastating for health, no matter how often you exercise – linked with early death, forms of cancer, obesity and type-2 diabetes – and older people are the most sedentary age group. Sixty minutes of daily exercise offsets the negative effects.

Stand with dignity

Mountain Pose (*Tadasana*), the starting
and reset position for yoga standing
postures, activates the lower body to
support your whole frame. It's also a
good practice when you feel a bit down
– feeling more aligned fosters a sense of
positivity, calmness and confidence.

1. Stand with feet shoulder-width apart,
outer edges parallel with each other (this
might look a little pigeon-toed). With your
arms and palms by your sides, press in
strongly to bring your whole body toward
the central line running from the top of
your head to your pelvic bone. Hold, then
relax, letting your shoulders drop.

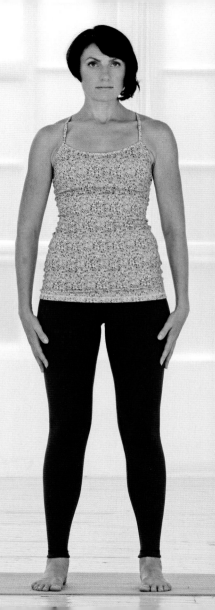

2. Rock forward and back on your feet, then from side to side until you find your centre. Lift your toes, spread them wide, keeping the base of the big toes firmly anchored, then replace each toe on the ground – try doing it one toe at a time, leaving space between each toe (it helps to spread your fingers, too). Firm your base diagonally by stretching from big toes to outer heels, and little toes to inner heels.

3. Activate the arches of your feet and lift up from there through your lower legs. Lift your thighs in order to raise your kneecaps, allowing the inner thighs to roll inward. Let your tailbone drop, as if you have a kangaroo tail weighing you down. As you exhale, lift the pelvic floor and draw your abdominal muscles up and back toward your spine. Feel the space you've made for the organs in your abdomen, and notice how secure they feel.

4. Lift up through both sides of the torso, drop your shoulders (imagine your shoulder blades descending) and extend the back of your neck. Feel your spine extending up and out of the pelvic bowl. Widen your collarbones and visualize your chest opening out from your breastbone like the pages of a book. Look forward, and imagine a thread at the crown of your head lifting you. Relax your jaw.

5. Hold the pose for a few minutes. As you exhale, feel your lower body descending down through your pelvis, legs, feet and into the floor. As you inhale, maintain that sense of grounding in your lower body while enjoying the upward lift in your chest and spine.

YOUR FRIEND THE WALL

The wall and the floor are there to help you toward good posture – there's a saying in the yoga world that the wall is your finest teacher – so use them both when exercising and as a posture check-in after periods of sitting. Feel the stability of the floor supporting you in a perfectly straight position when lying on your back, and practise standing with your heels, back of your pelvis and head touching a wall to experience what perfectly straight feels like.

The wisdom of the mountain

Old equates with strong, stable and wise in much world mythology. Table Mountain in Cape Town, South Africa, which stands prominent at the southernmost point of the African continent, has long been thought of as the Roman god Janus manifested. Janus is a sun deity depicted with two faces looking in opposite directions. He's associated with times of change and new beginnings – for example with new-year festivities – and is found sculpted over doorways and gates, often as an older man with a beard. He's vigilant, able to look at once right and left, inside and out, and to guard places of arrival and departure, making him a good archetype to contemplate as we reach the ends and beginnings of new decades. He was also commonly depicted on coins, representing communication and enterprise, and endeavours passing from one hand or generation to another.

When we stand tall in age we can feel better able to look in all directions and benefit from perspective. Equipped to look back to past decades and forward to those to come with poise and equanimity, we make better choices, allowing only useful things to travel forward with us and staying vigilant against less helpful information. Janus's insignia are the key that unlocks and the stick that beats away confusion and chaos.

RIGHT: Look for the head of Janus sculpted above gateways, entrances and other liminal spaces where worlds meet and possibilities branch.

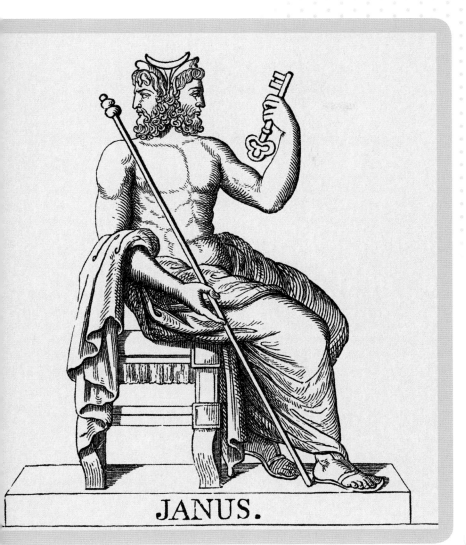

JANUS.

From the feet up

It's easier to maintain good posture if the feet are agile and sensitive to stimuli. Feeling in the feet declines with age, and around a third of people over 65 have trouble with painful or stiff feet. That makes it harder to stay active, move quickly and maintain a balanced body and gait. It also leads to that telltale "old-person" posture.

The feet are small compared with the impact of the bodyweight they have to absorb with each and every step. Putting on weight over the decades increases the load. Muscle tissue in the feet thins with age, tendons and ligaments fall out of balance, and the natural cushioning of fat beneath the heel and ball of the foot reduces. Nerves in the peripheries don't send messages as effectively to the brain, leading to loss in sensation, and blood can pool in the lower limbs, causing swelling. Joints stiffen if we don't put the feet through a good range of movement every day and the arches flatten, lengthening the feet. Bunions, hammer toes (stuck curled under) and other bone misalignments cause the feet to spread, meaning shoes no longer fit (wearing ill-fitting shoes probably caused the trouble in the first place).

One of the most useful things we can do to stay mobile is have our feet measured and wear properly supportive and well-fitting shoes – reportedly three out of four people over 65 wear shoes that are too small and people with diabetes are more likely to buy shoes that are wrong by at least half a size. It's simple to get measured and assessed at a running shop, and wearing the right shoes for the form of exercise you're doing is important. Shoes for racquet sports, for example, are designed to support the foot as it moves sideways and in stop-start movements, while running shoes offer more flexibility, and aerobics trainers have built-in cushioning to absorb impact.

TIP: Wear shoes indoors if you're nervous about falling – in one survey this seemed to reduce the likelihood of falls.

Grounding visualization

1. Stand barefoot and feel the four "corners" of each foot anchored to the floor: the base of your big and little toes, and both sides of your heels.

2. When you inhale, visualize the breath starting about a metre (three feet) beneath the earth, and with each exhalation imagine earthing any tension and nervous energy safely down into the ground.

3. To check your solidity, sway forward and back and from side to side until you find a point just forward from your heels at which you feel an effortless lift upward.

Dog-ball rolling

Specialist exercise balls used by chiropractors and bodyworkers are expensive; dog balls are cheap and just as good because they're small, and hard inside but flexible outside, which makes them comfortable as well as effective.

1. Stand up, take your bodyweight onto one foot and place the ball beneath your other foot. Roll the ball beneath your foot, very gently at first. Start carefully, noticing where your foot responds to the pressure and where you need to ease off. Work around the ball of the foot and the arch, down the inner and outer edges and the heel.

2. As you get more confident, press a little more firmly, but be careful – this feels so lovely that it can be easy to overdo it. Stop when you can't hold the pressure on the standing leg (this is also a great balance exercise). Repeat on the other foot.

3. Now try to lift the ball by grabbing it between your toes and the ball of the foot. This will be all-but impossible, but exercises the muscles that cause the toes to curl up with age. Do it several times with each foot.

Ankle and foot mobility sequence

This qigong sequence strengthens and mobilizes the ankles and boosts circulation to the feet.

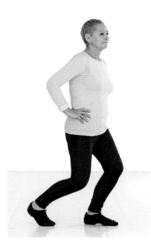

1. Stand with your feet hip-width apart, hands on your hips. Take a step back with your right foot and sink your weight into your left foot (keep the knee bent). Circle the right foot, keeping your toes on the ground, three times in one direction and then three times in the other. Feel the movement extending up into your hips. Repeat on the other leg.

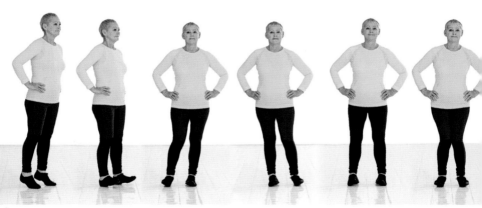

2. Return to the starting position, then rock forward onto your toes and back onto your heels. Repeat three times. Then rock from side to side three times. Notice if it's easier to move onto one side of the foot. Finally, rock to the outer edges of your feet and then the inner edges (bringing your knees together) three times.

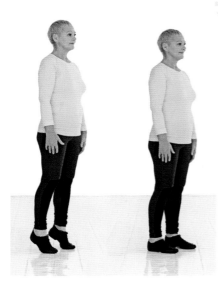

3. Come back to the starting position, release your hands from your hips and focus on your chest. Imagine there's a dot under each breast and another on your pubic bone, creating a triangle. Rising up onto your toes, imagine pressing the top two dots down to meet the bottom dot – this ballet trick engages your core muscles to keep you balanced. Hold for as long as you can remain balanced high on your tiptoes. Then drop your heels to the floor – you can use gravity to create a vibration through the body on landing if you enjoy that (but not if you have foot problems).

FOOT ACUPRESSURE AND MASSAGE

The acupressure point in the middle of the sole of the foot, called the Bubbling Spring in Traditional Chinese Medicine, is associated with bone health and growth, and is considered the wellspring of life. Also known as K1, it's the first and lowest point on the kidney meridian, and is found at the part of the foot that stays in contact with the ground during qigong, tai chi and yoga standing positions. When you walk or do a moving meditation practice (see page 324), take your focus here to root you to the energy of the earth.

Massage stimulates the nerves, increasing sensitivity in the feet, and boosts blood circulation, which is useful for the body's extremities as we age. It makes a good warm-up before exercise to loosen stiffness – rubbing the skin activates the fascia, helping to switch on balance (see page 82).

Foot self-massage

This qigong massage technique connects you to the grounding energy of the earth and calms the nervous system as it stimulates the first acupressure point on the kidney meridian.

1. Sit comfortably on the floor or on a chair and lift your right foot onto your left thigh, sole of the foot facing upward. Support the top of your foot with your left hand.

2. With the heel of your left hand make clockwise circles all over your foot, from the heel up to the base of the toes.

3. Now find the Bubbling Spring acupoint in the middle of the sole. It's at the base of the ball of the foot, between the pads – curl your toes in and you'll see an indentation where the point is. Circle around the point 36 times. As you do so, imagine the energy of the earth activating you at this point and welling up through your legs to the lower abdomen, where there's an energy centre that stores life force, the *dantien* (see page 90).

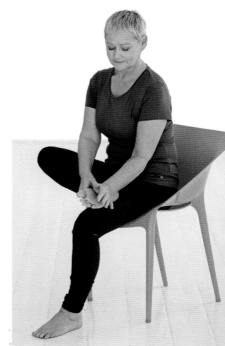

4. Change legs to repeat on the left foot using the heel of your right hand. If you would like to stimulate the kidney meridian channel further, stroke up a line from the inner ankle to the inside of the knee, up the inner thigh, then out over the top of the leg and around the hips to finish at the kidneys. Repeat on the other leg.

WINGS OF THE WOMB

Ayurveda, India's ancient health and longevity practice, connects the feet with the womb, since so many nerve endings in the foot channel into the pelvis. This makes foot exercise useful in the perimenopausal years to strengthen energy in the pelvic region and enhance confidence in your womanliness. Sit with your knees bent out to the sides and soles of the feet touching (in yoga this is the Bound Angle Pose, *Baddhakonasana*). Press your soles together strongly, then see if you can peel them apart like opening a book. Then, holding your ankles or knees, circle your upper body slowly. Start small, moving in time with your breath and making the rotation larger as you warm up. Feel the womb at the centre of your circle. Repeat in the other direction. If you find it hard to sit with feet together, cross them comfortably.

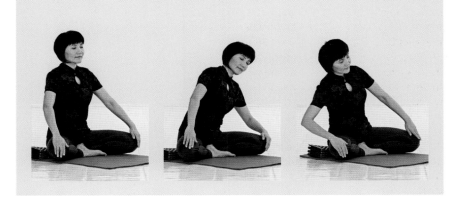

"All things are engaged in writing their history...Not a foot steps into the snow, or along the ground, but prints in characters more or less lasting, a map of its march. The ground is all memoranda and signatures..."

RALPH WALDO EMERSON

Find better balance

Once we reach 65 we're more likely to fall over. The WHO says falls are responsible for more than half the injury-related hospitalizations of people over 65 and account for 40 per cent of all deaths from injury, which increase exponentially with age. So protecting ourselves against falls – being better balanced – is one of the most useful things we can do to live longer, and to live well as we age.

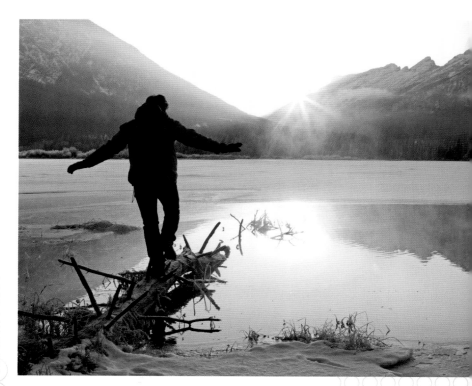

Falls have debilitating consequences not only in terms of pain and distress, which reduce quality of life, but also because they can lead to a loss of independence and confidence, which can stop us getting out and about. Fear of falling itself has been shown to lead to falls.

Exercising the balance – or vestibular – system is key to maintaining the even distribution of bodyweight we need to stay upright and on a steady footing. Proprioception is awareness of where the various parts of the body are in space; interoception is how we perceive our body from the inside, our internal map. Both help us maintain balance, and they change as our bodies shift with the decades. Injuries and illness, pregnancies and weight gain and loss all have an effect. Exercise, such as yoga, tai chi and qigong, enhances our awareness of where we are in space and sensitizes us to stimuli. Through practice we learn to make micro-adjustments that bring us back into balance and comfort. Since the fascia surrounding every part of the body contains masses of sensory receptors, training them in this way can be as effective in maintaining fitness as building muscle and bone, because it primes the body to regulate movement.

People with increased sensitivity to the body's sensory signals – from inside and out – seem to be able to use these gut feelings (or "viscerosensory information") to guide their movements and behaviour, so they make more effective decisions, particularly in situations that involve taking risks. Once we become more aware of our internal compass we can use it to orient ourselves, both in space and within the body.

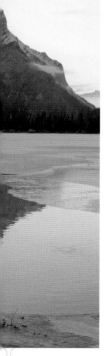

LEFT: Feeling brave enough to challenge your balance confidently is life-affirming and keeps the brain acting youthfully.

TIP: It's worth getting your eyes tested if you find it tricky to balance.

Test your self-awareness

This interoception exercise gives an indication of how focused your self-perception and sensory awareness are right now. Try repeating it before and after exercising to see how the activity connects disparate parts of the body. As you get used to the practice, tune inside while you go about your day, and try to detect your inner-body sensations amid the distractions of the outside world. How do the signals vary when you feel upset or unsteady and when you feel confident and sure-footed?

1. Stand with feet hip-width apart and close your eyes. Look inside your body. How far away are your feet from your head? Are your feet the same size or does one seem larger than the other? What about your hands? Maybe you have huge palms that seem to attach to your shoulders. Think about your head. Where do you feel it is in relation to your spine or shoulders?

2. Now turn your attention to the things you can't feel – the absences of perception. Can you feel one hip but not the other? Only one hand? Maybe you have no neck. Where are the gaps? What does that say about your body and your habits of movement and rest?

3. Where is the tension in your body? How do you visualize it? Where are you most comfortable inside? Which parts of your body do you trust? Which parts feel safe and which ones feel steady?

4. Before finishing, scan your body again and notice whether things have changed since you began the exercise.

"There is stillness even where there is movement. When there is movement there is stillness."

**SONG OF THE THIRTEEN TACTICS,
A CLASSIC TEXT OF TAI CHI**

Tai-chi balance training

Known as Wu Chi, this standing awareness position is used in preparation for practising the tai chi sequence. It brings increased awareness of the body in space and promotes balance by helping you switch on and feel the qualities of stability before starting to move.

1. Stand tall with your feet shoulder-width apart and slightly turned out. Let your arms relax by your sides. Then flex your hands so your palms face downward, but without being rigid. Look forward and soften your eyes by widening your gaze – imagine you are looking out through your temples. Relax your jaw.

2. Now close your eyes. Focus on your feet planted firmly on the earth and on your spine stretching upward. Feel how it is to be still but switched on, ready to move. Be aware, even when you are still, of the blood circulating inside the body, of the breath moving smoothly in and out. This stability is the beginning and ending of all movement.

GAZE POINT

Dancers use a single still point of focus to help them maintain balance and poise as they turn. In yoga, we bring the gaze, or *drishti*, to a fixed place as a way of concentrating focus and intensifying the practice. Test the effectiveness of this as you practise the Sun Salutation sequence (see page 64). When raising your arms, gaze at your thumbs; when bending forward, focus just beyond the tip of your nose; when looking up, gaze toward your third eye in the centre of your forehead (see page 339). In Downward Dog try to direct your gaze at your navel. Feel how this gives the practice more intention and balance, increases your awareness of the movements from the inside and disengages you from outside distraction. While fixing your gaze on a certain point outside the body increases stability, fixing it on the body itself brings an inward focus that feels even more centring.

Come back to centre

Imagine a plumb line that falls from the middle of the top of the head down the nose, chin, breastbone and spine, then drops through the pubic bone down to the inner knees and the point where the heels meet, a midline we draw toward and extend away from with each breath and every time we move. The body is symmetrical and for ideal alignment we should distribute our weight equally on both sides of the line.

The midline is the first function to develop when we are just a bunch of cells. In the beginning of the third week after conception, cells start to migrate to the centre of the bundle, forming a thicker ridge on either side of what is called the "primitive streak", around which the embryo forms. Cells then organize around this midline axis, including the beginnings

RIGHT: Visualize a line dropping from the top of your skull past your pubic bone and on down to the point between your feet, giving your body symmetry and balance.

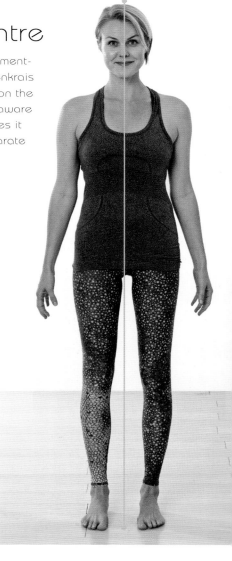

of the central nervous system, the skeleton and its associated muscles. Practitioners of Cranial Sacral Therapy believe that continuing to have a clarity of awareness of this midline is a sign of good health.

By practising yoga, tai chi or qigong we become better at consciously aligning ourselves around this central line. Yoga and traditional Chinese anatomy identify key energy points in the body along a central line aligned with the spine, including the point between the eyes, around the heart and at the solar plexus. Keeping these three areas aligned as we contract and expand the body in movement is thought to allow energy impulses to pass freely up and down the energy channel, which corresponds in conventional medicine to the positioning of the central nervous system.

In Traditional Chinese Medicine, the most important centre of balance along this line is at the *dantien*, located in the pelvis (see page 90). The pelvis is the body's physical centre of gravity when we stand. It's the fulcrum between the upper and lower body, the point of support around which we turn and pivot. When this area is stable and in balance, the spine can move freely and coordination between the legs and upper body flows freely.

In tai chi, dropping into a centred posture around the pelvis is valued for releasing stiffness and strain in the limbs, and bringing an ease to the body that allows us to coordinate movements and enter a state of relaxed readiness. In this position, like the centred Warrior (see page 40), we are prepared in body and mind to deal with attacks from any direction. In everyday life, that might be an uneven pavement or unexpected news rather than a ninja with a sword.

Awareness of the midline can feel very centring emotionally. At times when you feel scattered or disorientated, standing or lying down and visualizing a line running down through the body can bring a sense of order within life's chaos. It's a similar sensation to hugging your muscles toward the midline in yoga postures. The feeling of stability and support that brings to a pose is a comforting reminder as we age of how good it is to come back and orient ourselves around defining principles.

DANTIEN POWER

At the centre of the midline, about two fingers' width below the navel and right in the centre of your body mass, lies the most important energy centre in Traditional Chinese Medicine. Known as the *dantien*, it's the point at which everything comes into balance and the crucible in which energy is generated and stored. It's no coincidence that it's connected with the nourishing significance of the umbilicus. In the yoga system, this area corresponds to the *manipura* chakra, associated with self-esteem and confidence in yourself as a unique individual.

This area is used as a point of focus and balance in martial arts, but tuning in to it in any form of exercise can generate powerful feelings of strength, stability and the capacity to endure. When you need stamina, for example in the middle of a run or cycling up a hill, it can be useful to visualize each breath starting from this point.

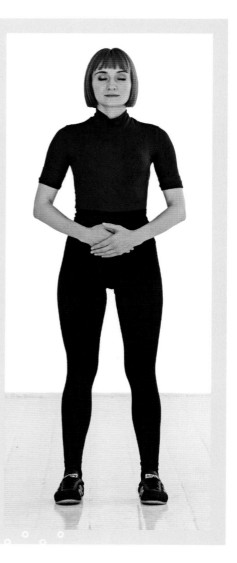

Central-line breathing

In this exercise you visualize the wave-like movement of the breath as your ribcage expands outward with the in-breath and contracts toward the midline as you exhale. It feels very grounding.

1. Start this simple breathing exercise lying on your back with legs stretched out or knees bent and feet flat on the floor. Make sure you're warm enough; it feels comforting to cover up with a warm blanket.

2. Close your eyes and bring your attention to your midline – trace it from the top of your head down your body and out between your legs, ending in the spot between your feet.

3. As you breathe in, imagine expanding out from that line – feel your ribcage widening equally on both sides of your chest, imagine your shoulders extending apart and your forehead flattening. Visualize your peripheries being nourished with freshly oxygenated blood.

4. As you breathe out, imagine everything drawing back in toward the midline, feeling your energy returning to centre. Sense a drawing in around your navel and a focus of attention around your third-eye area in the centre of your forehead (see page 339).

5. Repeat for up to five minutes, enjoying the expansion on the in-breath and the grounding sense of returning to centre on the out-breath. Return to your natural rhythm of breathing before rolling over and slowly getting up.

Find your centre

This exercise brings awareness of the pelvis as a fulcrum – it's easier to sense this when the pelvis is in contact with the floor. Once you've learned the basics of the movement with the support of the floor, start to notice the position of the pelvis when you are standing, bending, lifting and carrying. This helps support the spine and internal organs. In this exercise keep the movements slow and smooth and your jaw and forehead relaxed.

1. Lie on your back with knees bent and feet flat on the floor, hip-width apart. The outer edges of your feet should be parallel with each other – you may need to move your heels out slightly. Relax your head and shoulders comfortably and rest your hands either on your belly or by your sides, palms up. Notice which parts of your back are in contact with the floor, and which areas feel tense and which relaxed.

2. On an exhalation, press your lower back into the floor. As you inhale, let it lift away. Repeat a number of times – as you exhale, notice how your stomach muscles contract and how your navel moves toward your spine when your pelvis tilts up, lower back flattening against the floor.

3. As you inhale, notice how the tops of your thighs drop toward the floor and your lower back lifts. Repeat this

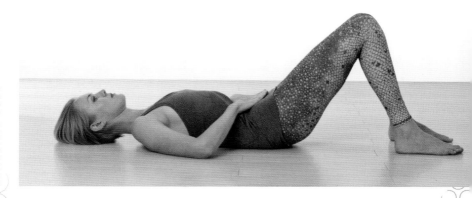

hollowing and tilting action, coordinating it with your inhalations and exhalations. Notice how your head and shoulders join the movement quite naturally.

4. Now exhaling, lift your right hip slightly by pressing into the floor with your right foot. Notice your abdominal muscles contract on that side. Inhale and relax the back of your pelvis to the ground. Exhaling again, repeat on the left hip. Set up a slow rocking from side to side.

5. Imagine your pelvis is a clock – 6 o'clock is at your tailbone and 12 at your lower back; 3 o'clock is on your left hip and 9 on your right. Find the centre of the clock. Rock your pelvis up to 12 o'clock while

exhaling, and inhale back to 6. Repeat, feeling the imprint of your pelvis on the floor, as if you were using an inked printing block; try to keep the pressure even to print the picture evenly. Now rock sideways from 3 to 9 o'clock, again keeping the pressure even across your sacrum.

6. Finally, circle around the clock five times in one direction and five in the other. Focus on the areas where you find it tricky to keep the pressure even. Come to rest back at centre. Does your back feel different from when you started the exercise? Maybe the movements have freed up tension in the shoulders or hips. Roll to one side and push on your hands to sit up.

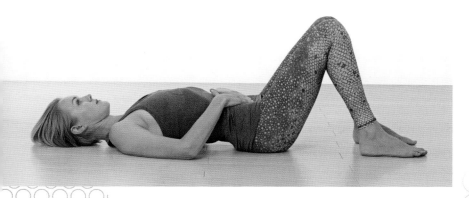

Hugging to the midline

This muscular action, taught in Anusara Yoga, ensures you engage your core muscles in order to move safely and with security – the core being all the muscles that support your frame, not just those around the abdomen.

1. Start standing. To learn the action, stretch your arms out from the shoulders, palms facing forward, so the little-finger side of your hand is parallel with the floor. Stretch them out as far as you can extend your fingers. Feel your shoulder blades pull apart.

2. Now, maintaining the stretch, slide your arm bones back, feeling the shoulder blades pull together and the head of the arm bones engage into the joints. Feel how stable and supported your arms feel now. This is the feeling to aim for when exercising: drawing the arms and legs (and head) in toward the inner muscles of the torso supports the peripheral parts of the body – those most prone to injury.

3. Now hug in your outer shins and thighs, pull in the sides of your body to support your hips, slide your shoulder blades toward each other and down toward your lower back, and draw the bottom of the ribcage back toward the spine. Imagine drawing the skin to the muscle, and the muscle to the bone. This physical integration – the bringing of the outer to the inner – has a stabilizing and calming effect on the mind, making us feel more focused, contained and safe, both when still and in movement. A hug is always comforting!

Yoga tree balance

It's easy to try too hard when practising yoga balances and to get fixated on not wobbling or falling over, when moving into a pose with softness can be more effective, especially for balancing postures. This moving version of Tree Pose (*Vrksasana*) challenges us not to care, while teaching how to trust the inner support of the core. Using inner strength is more effective in maintaining balance than extending your limbs at the peripheries.

1. Stand with feet hip-width apart and close your eyes. Sense down into your feet and the stability of the four corners of your soles: the base of the big and little toes and the outer and inner edges of your heels. Feel your pelvis aligned over your feet, and your shoulders over your hips.

2. Open your eyes and shift your bodyweight over your right foot. Lift your other foot off the ground and rest it above your

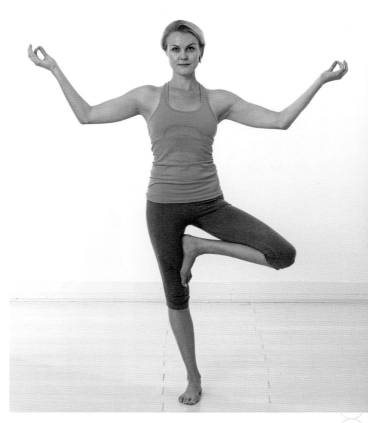

ankle or above your knee. If you're flexible, pick it up and rest it at the top of your standing leg – there's a little ledge at the top of the thigh. Press the sole of the raised foot into the standing leg and, pushing back, feel the resistance. Imagine screwing in wing nuts on either side of your hips to keep them pinned in. Put your hand on a wall for balance if you need to. Extend your arms out to the side with your elbows bent, and touch your thumbs to your index fingers to increase your sense of security. Feel how that helps you draw your shoulder blades together.

3. Now play with the pose. How far can you tilt your torso to the left, taking your left elbow toward the raised knee? Relax your jaw and extend your arms further if it helps. Try focusing on a fixed spot in front of you, but don't be afraid to fall over – see how far you can take the bend. Then curve in the other direction.

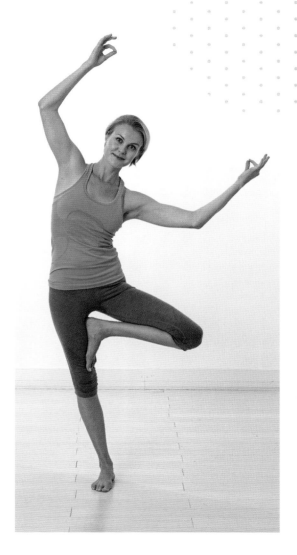

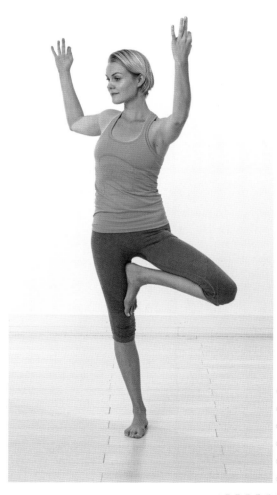

4. Come back to centre. Breathe in to stretch up, then breathe out to twist your torso to the right, away from your bent knee. Start the twist in your lower abdomen – can you feel how this engages your core muscles? Again, don't be afraid to topple. Return to the centre and revolve to the left on an out-breath. Take a few calm breaths in and out and then come back to centre.

5. Place your raised foot on the floor, close your eyes and sense both halves of your body. Do they feel different? Can you articulate why? Once you feel centred, repeat to the other side.

Deity of balance

As our hormones shift in the mid-years, so the mix of what makes our bodies male and female alters. This can be such a downer in terms of self-awareness and body-confidence and yet useful because it forces us to rethink the way we relate to our bodies and their physical shape and functioning. It raises such fascinating questions. What makes us male or female? Are we still female if our female hormones are diminished? Are we female if we have no womb? How can we have the confidence to do a body scan in a meditation or yoga class when our bodies no longer fit the patterns of ourselves that we have settled into over decades? We've probably not had to think this much about ourselves and our shifting shape since puberty or pregnancy.

Archetypes can make useful body-contemplation aids at this time, and help us explore feelings that are hard to put into words or for which habitual expressions aren't helpful. Our changing physiology has a powerful effect on our emotions and mental wellbeing, and new ways of thinking can help rein in the uncontrollable discomfort that comes from a mismatch between how we once saw ourselves and where we are now.

From the Hindu pantheon comes the deity Ardhanarisvara, who represents godhead in its male and female forms in a single body. In depictions, the right half of the body is male (Shiva) and the left female (Shakti, in the form of Shiva's consort Parvati) – because godhead manifests and honours feminine and masculine energy equally. The divine quality of this balancing of traditional gender qualities can be helpful to keep in mind for its positivity and for the potential offered by non-duality and dynamic balance. Shifting hormones make room for new and perhaps more adventurous ways of being.

RIGHT: Ardhanarisvara – the Sanskrit word *ardha* means "half" – epitomizes male and female energies meeting at the midline of the body in perfect balance.

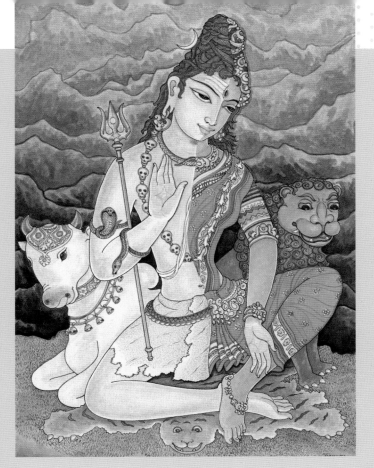

"Unified am I, quite undisturbed. Unified is my soul, unified is my eye, unified is my ear, unified is my breath, in and out; undisturbed is my diffusive breath. Unified, quite undisturbed, is the whole of me."

ATHARVA VEDA, THE VEDIC TEXT OF PROCEDURES FOR EVERYDAY LIFE

A balanced temperature

Sudden hot flushes are the most common symptom of menopause – three out of four women experience them and they can recur on and off for years, even decades. The causes aren't proven, but hormonal imbalance is probably the main one.

Overheating is one of the most obvious signs of a system out of balance. Usefully, flushes are impossible to ignore, which counter-intuitively makes them actually quite helpful, forcing us to pay attention to ourselves and look at different ways of engaging the body and changing the way we live to build in more rest and reduce stress; both seem to help ease the symptoms.

Useful self-help remedies include herbal preparations (see page 240) and cutting back on trigger foods and drink. Alcohol is thought to be one, because by dilating blood vessels it directs blood to the surface of the skin, making you warmer; caffeine works in a similar way by significantly promoting blood flow.

Obvious ways of cooling the body quickly, such as cold showers, cool packs and sprays, make helpful fire-fighting strategies. Longer term, Ayurveda recommends *pitta*-reducing measures – *pitta* is the subtle energy governing the body's inner fire and so also digestion, metabolism and energy-production (see page 17). *Pitta*-reducing plans include

cooling foods (see page 259), the Cooling Breath technique recommended to reduce body temperature and diffuse anger (see page 102), and Alternate Nostril Breath (*Nadi Shodhana Pranayama*) to cultivate more equilibrium (see page 344). Many women find the refreshing effects of restorative yoga poses useful, too – they bring about a deep sense of calm and wellbeing and include supported Corpse Pose (*Savasana*, see page 385) and Yoga Nidra (see page 154).

Conversely, some women find a vigorous, heating yoga practice (such as ashtanga or hot yoga) extremely useful for burning off excess heat – they report that it seems to regulate the system for a few days. For example, when practised at the weekend, it can stave off symptoms into the week. A University of Granada study of 200 previously sedentary postmenopausal women found that exercise helped them manage hot flushes while improving their general fitness, cardiovascular health and overall wellbeing.

Energetically, heat shares the positive as well as the negative qualities of fire –

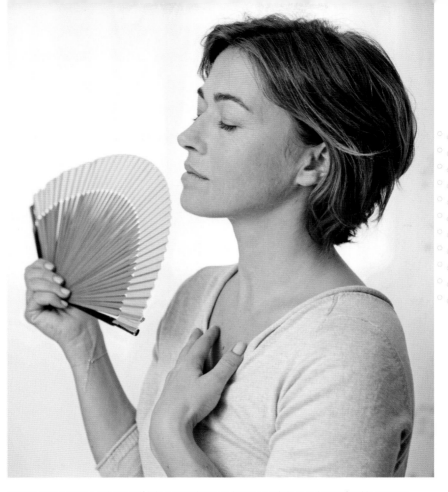

ABOVE: Deep breathing and other self-help stress-reduction techniques may help to cool uncomfortable symptoms.

it transforms as it consumes, leading to greater clarity and an opportunity for new beginnings. If we pass through and survive the inner fire, welcoming it as an opportunity to burn away those things that are no longer useful, then we might emerge with new vision and intentions.

Cooling breath *(Sitali Pranayama)*

1. Sit comfortably with an upright spine and take a few moments to tune in to your breathing. Just watch it moving in and out. Then stick your tongue out and try to curl up the sides to make a little tube. (Don't worry if you can't do this – genetically some of us can't. Instead, open your mouth slightly and rest the tip of your tongue on the ridge behind your upper teeth.)

2. Breathe in very slowly through the "straw" of your rolled tongue (or open mouth), listening to the soft hissing sound. Hold the cool breath as long as feels comfortable, then exhale through your nose, relaxing your tongue and mouth. Repeat three to five times, then relax.

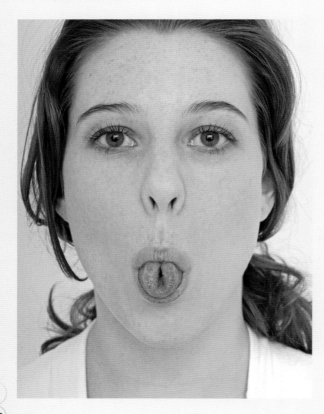

Reclining bound angle pose *(Supta Baddhakonasana)*

This restorative yoga posture promotes blood flow to the pelvic region, and is recommended to relieve menopausal symptoms, including overheating. To bring a nurturing focus to the womb and ovaries, you might like to place your hands on your lower abdomen in Yoni Mudra, with index fingers together and thumb tips touching to create a triangle shape. Rest the tips of the index fingers on your pubic bone and your thumbs on your belly. You will need two yoga bolsters, a blanket and an eye pillow.

1. Place one bolster horizontally and the other vertically on top into a T-shape. Fold the blanket into a long sausage. Sit with your buttocks in front of the sloping bolster and lean back, so your head rests on the highest point and your sacrum is supported by the end of the bolster.

2. Sit up and bring the soles of your feet together. Wrap the middle of the blanket roll over your feet, pulling it in under your ankles and passing the ends behind your knees and outer thighs, bunching them up to support the weight of your legs.

3. Lie back over the bolster, feeling your back and head well supported. Place the eye pillow gently over your eyes. Relax your arms by your sides, palms facing up. Once you are fully comfortable, settle into the pose for between five and ten minutes. Cover yourself with a blanket if you feel cold. If you feel stressed, come out of the pose or rearrange the supports.

4. Remove the eye pillow, push down with your hands and try to sit up, leading with your chest. Use your hands to pull your knees together gently.

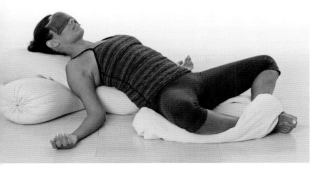

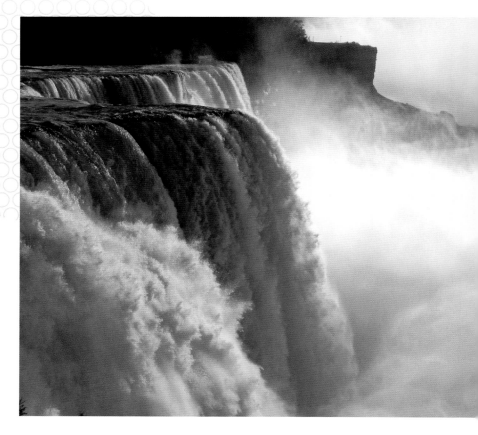

Water therapy

The medicinal powers of water are championed by hydrotherapists for balancing internal heat in the body. Water therapy acts on body temperature, working with the constriction and dilation of blood vessels (as do hot flushes).

Devised by Father Sebastian Kneipp in the late 19th century, the system is based on self-care techniques using water application to restore balance to the body systems. He recommended it specifically to counter the effects of ageing.

LEFT: In a study at Baylor University, women who visualized an image associated with coolness during a relaxation session – most often a waterfall or rain shower – reported a dramatic decrease in hot flushes.

How does it work? A warm bath dilates the blood vessels, increasing blood flow away from the internal organs and toward the surface of the skin. Improved circulation benefits the tissues (better delivery of oxygen and nutrients) and boosts the immune and waste-cleansing systems, while the warmth of the water relaxes the muscles.

When skin is exposed to cool water, blood vessels narrow, directing blood away from the surface to protect the internal organs, which has a stimulating effect. Sports therapists know the value of cryotherapy, or post-workout ice baths, to reduce swelling and fluid build-up, provide instant pain relief by numbing nerve endings, and drain lactic acid from overworked muscles to relieve soreness. Cold water seems to kick-start the immune system, too, boosting numbers of disease-fighting white blood cells. Moving between hot and cold water stimulates the production of endorphins, the body's natural opiates, and the greater the variance in temperature, the more invigorating the effect, hence the euphoria of a dash out from a sauna into a pool of icy water or snow.

TONIC FOR HOT FLUSHES

Traditionally, twice-weekly cold sitz baths help with hot flushes (a sitz bath is a hip bath). Basically, you sit in a plastic bowl of tepid water for 30 seconds to 3 minutes, ideally with the water reaching from upper thigh to mid-abdomen. Kneipp recommends this before bed to cure heat-induced insomnia, or in the morning if you wake from a soaked night feeling tired and unrefreshed.

Both hot and cold water can be useful for hot flushes. Cold water seems the most obvious way to reduce body temperature – run wrists under a cold tap or spritz the face with a water spray kept in the fridge for instant refreshment. For the most effective cooling shower, start with the water warm, gradually turning it colder as you run a hand-held spray over your face and then your limbs, working down the body for 30 seconds. A short (few seconds to two minutes) cool bath is also useful – hydrotherapists recommend a temperature of 10–24°C (50–75°F). Rub dry briskly or put on dry clothes (linen is best) over damp skin and walk or exercise for 15 minutes, until you reach normal body temperature.

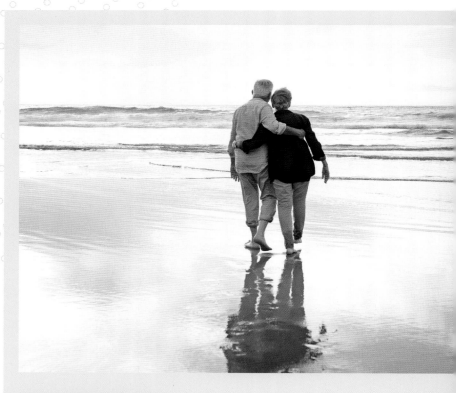

REINVIGORATE YOUR FEET

A cold footbath first thing in the morning and before bed (fill a bucket to the calves and tread in the water for one to three minutes) is valued for drawing down heat from the head and upper body or dealing with fatigue brought on by a day's work in hot conditions. Alternatively, put on a pair of damp cotton socks, then cover them with dry woollen socks and go to bed (leave on for half an hour).

If you have access to a stream, pool or the sea, all the better for paddling in water up to your calves. Kneipp also recommends

Be aware that cold-water therapies can promote warming – the initial blast of cold directs circulation away from the skin, but when it stops, blood heads out again to the peripheries, which can feel warming. A longer warm bath (30–35°C/85–95°F) might help more, by relaxing the muscles and reducing the stress response as well as improving blood circulation. This is recommended before bed.

> "All wish to be healthy and live long, but few do something about it."
>
> **FATHER SEBASTIAN KNEIPP**

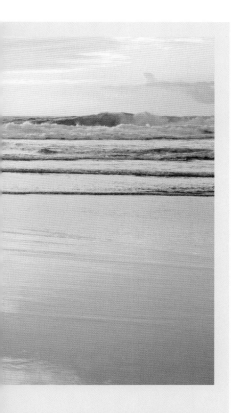

ABOVE: Walking the seashore barefoot with a loved one is a tonic for heart and mind as well as rejuvenating for the feet.

walking barefoot over dew-soaked grass, on wet stones or even in new-fallen snow, to harden and brace the system. Not for the faint-hearted!

COLD-WATER CARE

In a study, 59 out of 60 women completing the first trial into Kneipp hydrotherapy for menopausal symptoms – they applied two sessions of self-care daily using cold water – expressed a strong interest in continuing the cold stimuli after the trial ended.

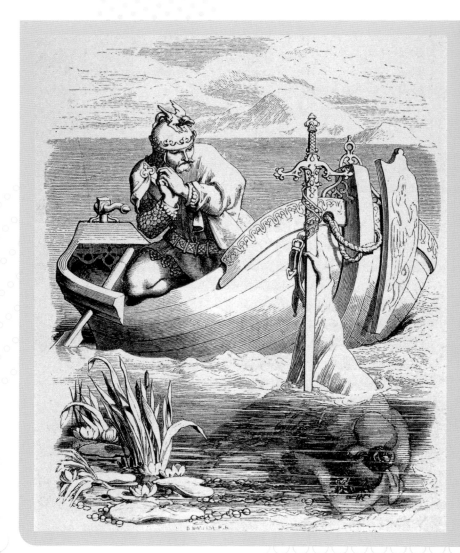

Water of eternal life

Bodies of water are associated with rejuvenation and extended life in many traditions – not least with the promise of eternal life offered by the holy sacrament of Christian baptism. It's often a female association. In China, the well is linked with the life-giving properties of the womb, while female deities stand guard over lakes and pools around the globe, from the Romano-British Sulis Minerva in Bath to the rusalka of Slavic legend. This fierce Lady Luck requires propitiation with coins and precious-metal votives because she decides whether to bless and grant wishes with her powers or to harm and cast curses. The Lady of the Lake offers up the enchanted sword Excalibur but also bleeds Merlin of his magic, leaving him impotent. There's a metaphor for ageing!

Perhaps the most potent symbol of watery female power – to rebirth, to curse, to bless – is the cauldron, a womb-shaped container presided over by older women with the knowledge and experience to transform lowly ingredients into a source of inspiration and rejuvenation. In the Welsh tradition, the greatest treasure of the kingdom of King Bran, told of in *The Mabinogion*, is the Cauldron of Rebirth, which has the power to regenerate and restore to strength. For this reason, it is associated with great wisdom, including secret knowledge of worlds beyond our own. In her own cauldron of inspiration, so the bard Taliesin tells us, the enchantress Ceridwen concocts a brew that will confer on whoever drinks it the mysteries of knowledge and inspiration; just three drops of this "charmed liquor" give the gift of foresight and the ability to change form at will.

LEFT: The Lady of the Lake presents King Arthur with the magical weapon Excalibur, which comes from another realm and must be returned there when Arthur dies.

Hot springs, long life

In many parts of the world where naturally heated volcanic water springs out of the earth – Japan, Iceland, France, Italy – longevity has been attributed to regular bathing in those waters. Legend has it that people became aware of the curative powers of the waters by watching injured animals approach the springs for healing. Sulphur springs especially are associated with longevity, and people head to them from across the globe, now as in centuries past, to calm skin conditions and respiratory disorders and ease joint pain, as well as problems of the liver and of the digestive system, by bathing in the sulphur-rich water or mud or partaking of vapour inhalations. Our bodies need sulphur (for heart function and metabolism, flexible joints and cartilage and healthy skin) and it's true that places where it occurs abundantly in the soil and inland waters (Iceland and Japan) tend to be associated with long life, but there's no good evidence to support how it might work.

That said, balneotherapy – the medicinal use of mineral-rich thermal waters – is a very old therapy that is still very much alive. Mesolithic finds show us that natural springs have been places of pilgrimage in Europe since 5000 BCE. Their healing powers are mentioned in the Bible and in Egyptian texts, and Roman soldiers used *salus per aquam* (or spa, "health through water") as a restorative after fighting in battle, as did Montezuma centuries later on another continent.

Today hundreds of mineral spas are licensed for curative use in the French and German medical systems, and the wellness spa industry is booming. What we can prove, of course, is the longevity of this water, thought to have fallen some 5–10,000 years ago – a time when the land was forested and we'd just started farming and forming settlements. Over those thousands of years these drops of rain trickled hundreds of metres (or feet) down through the bedrock beneath us to be warmed by the earth's crust before springing up once more, bubbling to the surface through a crack or fissure to begin the water cycle all over again.

RIGHT: We have always sought purification, healing and solace in naturally heated waters that bubble up from the earth's core.

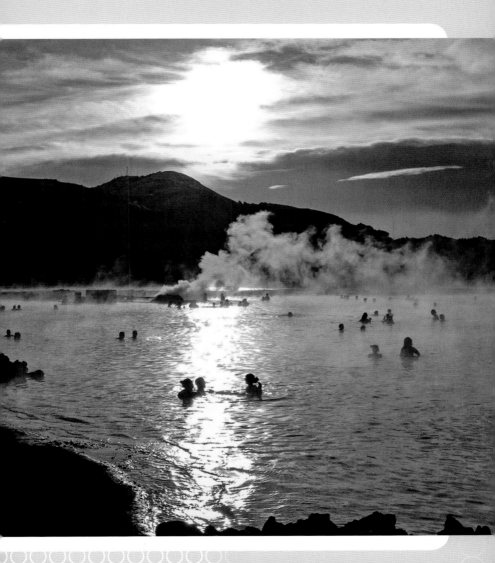

Support from the inside

As we get older it's common to feel that everything's heading southward and gravity is taking a toll, not just on the face and skin but on our internal organs. This is especially true for women in the genital area and urinary tract.

The organs and muscles in this area contain oestrogen receptors. Oestrogen has an uplifting effect, so when that starts to wane in the perimenopausal period, connective tissue and muscles in the pelvic area can become both weaker and stiffer – less supportive – and the sensory threshold of the bladder is raised. Up to 40 per cent of postmenopausal women are thought to suffer from pelvic-organ prolapse or stress/"urge" urinary incontinence.

Postural stress exacerbates the feeling of the organs dragging. The effort of prolonged standing in particular adds to the stress of pregnancy and birth, of chronic coughing and of carrying extra weight – all weaken the support system that holds everything nicely in place.

In most cases, lifestyle changes can really help – more exercise, better posture, stopping smoking and eating plenty of vegetables, fruit and wholegrains to prevent the straining that comes with constipation.

Exercises that contract and release the muscles of the vaginal wall (see opposite) bring more tone to the pelvic muscles, abdomen and lower back, but maintaining good posture is also vital – play with the Find your Centre clock exercise (see page 92) to establish a position in which your pelvic organs feel light and supported. It's likely to be when you have an inward curve in the lower back that tilts the pelvis into the 6 o'clock position. When you're standing, this allows the pelvic organs to rest above, and supported by, the pelvic bones. Put it into action as you move around, and actively pull your abdominal muscles up and back as you breathe out. This is especially important when lifting and carrying.

TIP: Activating the feet really helps to lift the pelvic area. Practise the Stand with Dignity exercise (see page 74), sensing how you can guide the uplift that starts in the arches of the feet up the insides of your legs and up to the lower abdomen.

Pelvic-floor squeeze and release

This yoga exercise uses the power of the breath and the naturally occurring uplift as we exhale to work the muscles that support the torso and internal organs. Unlike regular pelvic-floor exercises, it puts equal emphasis on relaxing the muscles: hard, stiff muscles don't work as well as toned but relaxed muscles. Avoid if you are menstruating.

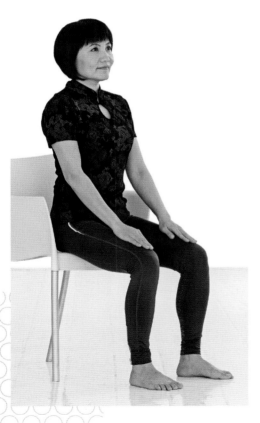

1. Sit comfortably on the floor or on a chair with your spine upright and your pelvic floor well supported by the floor or seat. Close your eyes and watch your breath moving in and out. After tuning in to a few breaths, watch what happens at the end of the out-breath – can you sense a slight lift in the muscles of the vagina? Watch how it releases downward as you breathe in and your pelvic floor feels supported again by the floor or seat.

2. Now, at the end of the next out-breath, try to harness that natural lift and actively squeeze the walls of the vagina in and up. Lift as far as feels comfortable. As you inhale, release the tension, let go of the muscles and enjoy the support of the floor again. Repeat for a few rounds, lifting on the out-breath and releasing on the in-breath.

Moving bridge pose

A dynamic variation of the yoga Bridge Pose (*Setubandha Sarvangasana*), this works the abdominal and pelvic muscles while demonstrating how to start a pelvic uplift in the feet. The slower you do this exercise, the stronger the effect. It can be helpful to practise with a yoga block (or two) between the thighs – squeeze to keep the block firmly in place as you lift and lower to help you locate the support the inner thighs provide for the pelvic organs. It's also lovely to align your breathing with your movements.

1. Lie on your back with knees bent and feet flat on the floor, shoulder-width apart and with the outer sides of your feet parallel with each other or with the sides of a yoga mat.

2. As you breathe in, reach your arms up to vertical and push into your feet to start lifting your pelvis. Continue stretching your arms back behind your head and lift up onto tiptoes if that feels good. If it compresses the lower back, keep your feet down and your hips low.

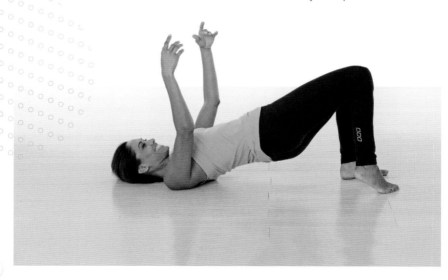

3. Release on the out-breath, bringing your arms back beside your torso and releasing your back very slowly from the upper spine down. Tuck your tailbone under to extend your spine as you try to lower vertebra by vertebra, tailbone last.

4. Repeat for up to three minutes. Notice how the lift starts in the feet and how pressing into the ground sets off a reaction that lifts the pelvic muscles. As you practise, think about how you can transfer this understanding to upright situations, and how you can use the heels and balls of the feet to bring a lift to your pelvic muscles and posture each time you exhale.

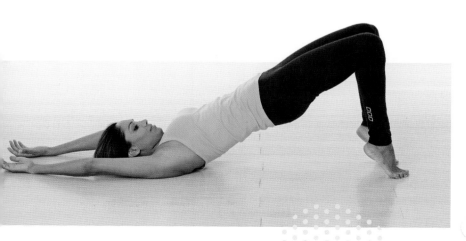

Expand laterally

After the age of 30 in men and 40 in women we lose our range of mobility in the sides of the body unless we actively practise lateral stretching – not a movement we tend to do much in everyday life.

The largest study of flexibility – with 6,000 participants – found that the trunk and shoulders in particular became less mobile and are most affected by ageing. Elbows and knees remained relatively mobile in comparison, because of the way we routinely use our bodies. If we don't put a part of the body through its full range of movement most days, it loses flexibility at an accelerated rate. It's known as "age decay". In women, age decay is significantly slower than in men, and this advantage progressively increases with age. Lack of flexibility has been linked with falls in older people, perhaps because it stops us recovering in time when we lose balance.

However, only about half of the variability in flexibility is explained by age. If we adopt an active lifestyle as a young adult and then increase that activity into middle age and beyond, the good news is that we can continue to enjoy a full range of movement in the sides of the body (and other non-habitually used muscles). This is not so for joints, such as the knees and elbows, which already get put through a wide range of motion most days.

Primal movement

This is a great way to regain a more natural range of motion throughout the body. It's a series of movements based on observations of animals and especially our primate forebears. It works around movement patterns that replicate the type of activity our ancestors would have done 40 generations ago – hanging, sprinting, squatting, crawling, rolling, twisting, jumping and so on. These total-body movements result in all-over body strength and capacity rather than the kind of bulging biceps that single-focus workouts tend to promote – think of the distance runner with well-developed legs but a stiff back and weedy arms.

Movements based on child development can also be incredibly helpful in mobilizing parts of the body we don't habitually use (particularly stiff shoulders and hips and a trunk that doesn't rotate easily), and in rehabilitation after injury. Similar to primal training, they take us back to elemental movements of the human body, such as pushing up to look over one shoulder – that cute thing babies do, which eventually leads

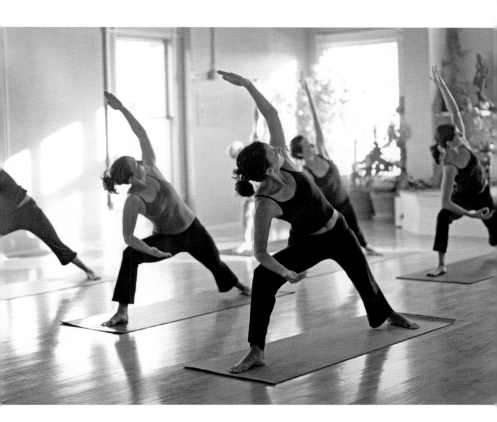

to rolling onto their backs. The rotation involved in pushing up from lying on your front to look behind one shoulder is especially helpful in realigning the trunk, stabilizing the core and relieving stiff joints. Other useful developmental movement exercises include Happy Baby (see page 119), crawling and spiral-patterned twists.

ABOVE: Lateral stretching, from the outer edge of the foot to the fingertips, forms part of the traditional sequence of standing poses in yoga.

TIP: To try out primal movement, look for "foundational", "functional" or "animal pattern" classes.

WHY CRAWLING IS GOOD

In *As You Like It* Shakespeare describes the seven ages of man (see page 20). He says the last stage of life is "second childishness" – so let's make the most of that, starting with learning to crawl again. This is an important action for the body, part of human hardwiring that helps us develop pathways between the right and left sides of the brain and body, as well as hand–eye coordination. The cross-patterning of our limbs diagonally with their opposites is key to total body coordination and teaches the hips and shoulders how to work together efficiently. It builds the core strength you need to take your extremities in to the centre and out again, knitting everything together. Crawling also gently builds the essential or "reflexive" strength we need for good balance and proprioception, awareness of the body in space. You can practise crawling with your knees on the floor – gentle pressure on the kneecaps helps build cartilage and, on the wrists, increases strength – or with your knees just hovering off the floor to build a strong core while releasing tension in the joints.

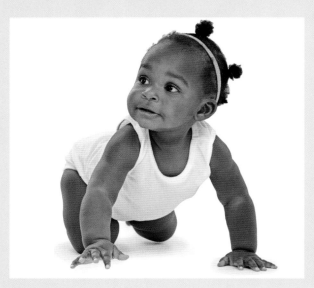

LEFT: Maintaining the movement patterns of a child helps us feel young: with practice we can retrain body and brain into easier ways of getting around.

Happy baby *(Ananda Balasana)*

A brilliant hip-opener, this replicates a position we all adopt as babies. Once you get used to the pose, start to move in it, pulling down on each foot in turn to set up a comforting rocking action. This feels great on the sacrum.

1. Lie on your back and bring your legs toward your chest. Reach around the inside of each leg with each arm and grasp your feet (hold the instep or heels if you can). Your lower legs should be perpendicular to the floor and your feet flat, facing the ceiling. Pull your knees down toward your armpits.

2. Hold the pressure on your feet and relax your head and shoulders on the floor. If the stretch feels easy, press into your sacrum to take the base of your spine nearer the ground. Rest in the pose for up to three minutes, following your breath and pressing your knees down with the out-breath. Rock from one side to the other if that feels good. Roll to one side and rest there for a moment before pushing up.

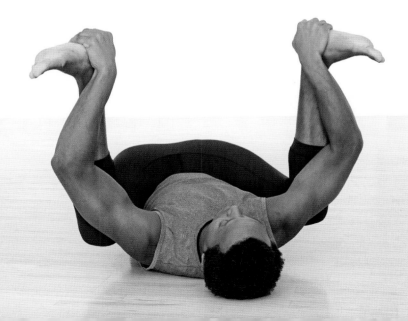

Crescent moon stretch

This pose feels easy because you're lying on the floor, but the long lateral stretch extends all the way up the side of the body from the thighs through the abdominal oblique muscles to the armpits, making it incredibly effective in opening up the sides of the body.

1. Lie on your back with your legs straight. Raise your head to look down your body and check that everything's in line and then lower it to the ground again. Breathing in, raise your arms overhead and lower them to rest behind your head if possible. Take your left wrist with your right hand and curve to the right. Make sure both shoulders stay on the floor; come back to centre if you've gone a little too far.

2. Now walk your feet to the right, making a crescent-moon shape with your body. Only go as far as feels comfortable. Feel your left buttock heavy on the floor, and if you're still comfortable, rest your left ankle on your right ankle.

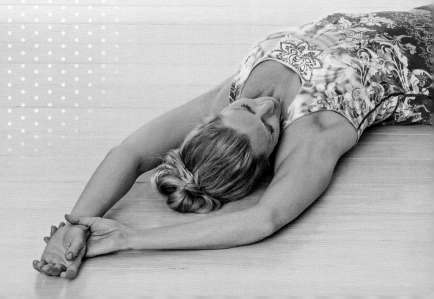

3. Relax in the stretch for up to five minutes. Savour the lengthening from your ankle up the side of your body to your wrist, and the corresponding compression on your right side. Breathe into your belly and soften your shoulders – draw them down away from your ears. Relax your jaw and forehead and soften your gaze.

4. When you're ready, uncross your ankles and walk your feet back to centre. Release your wrist and come back to alignment. Lie quietly and notice how different your stretched side feels. Repeat to the left.

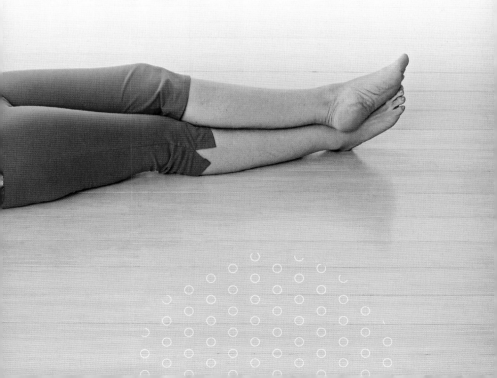

Gate pose *(Parighasana)* flow

This flowing sequence eases you into lateral stretching by twisting and mobilizing the trunk. This frees the area around the ribcage, which often gets "stuck" as we age, and helps to make deep breathing easier.

1. Kneel up (on a folded blanket if preferred) and stretch out your right leg, keeping the foot in line with your left knee. Either keep the foot on the floor or rest the ball of your foot on a yoga block if your calf is tight. Take your left arm out to the left and place the palm on the floor (or a yoga block) in line with your knee. Lift your right arm and cup the back of your skull with your right hand.

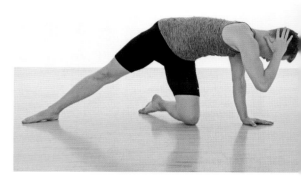

2. Breathing in, revolve your torso upward, taking the weight of your head in your top hand. Let your elbow point skyward and look up. Exhaling, revolve back down to the starting position. Open and close a few times, starting the twist in your lower abdomen. Feel the top ribs spiralling back and the lower ribs softening forward. Breathe into the back of your top lung in the extended position.

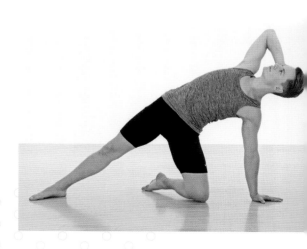

3. When you feel ready, release your top hand in the upward-facing position and lengthen it over your head; look up if you can. Feel the stretch from the outer edge of your outstretched foot to the tips of your fingers. To increase the stretch, breathe smoothly in and out and lift from right ankle to right knee, lift the right thigh, feel the intercostal muscles between your ribs opening up, enjoy the opening in your armpit and lengthen from upper arm to fingertips – don't let your arm be floppy.

4. Release the arm, draw in the outstretched leg and sit on your heels. Feel the difference in the sides of your body, hips and shoulders, before repeating to the other side.

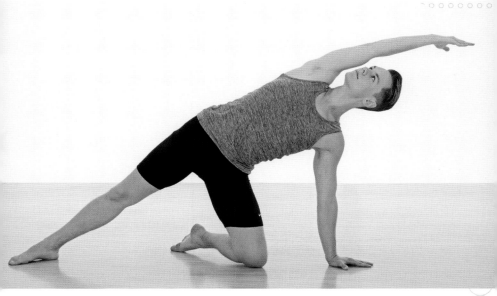

A pain-free back

The health of the spine is key to continuing movement and agility. Joseph Pilates believed that we're as old as our spinal column, and considered people with a stiff spine in their 30s "old", and those with mobile spines at 60 "young". The lower back can prove particularly problematic as we age. This is the part of the spine that's most mobile, so if other areas of the spine stiffen, this area absorbs the strain, leading to increased risk of injury.

Chronic lower-back pain is the most common health problem resulting in disability in people over 60. That age group is more likely to suffer lower-back pain than younger adults – 65–85 per cent of older people report musculoskeletal pain and up to 70 per cent of that is in the back. Women are seemingly twice as susceptible as men. Back pain often goes unreported to doctors – we stoically live with it – and there's evidence that we become better at living with pain as we get older. Studies using heat as a stimulus suggest there's an age-related increase in pain threshold, as the parts of the brain responsible for pain-processing reduce with age.

As well as being under-reported, persistent lower-back pain is also under-managed and treated by doctors and in nursing homes because it's hard to diagnose the causes – in the majority of cases there's no obvious pathology and pain may be the result of problems elsewhere in the skeleton. In any case, lower-back pain is a reliable predictor of depression and anxiety, and a key factor in repeated falls.

If life becomes increasingly sedentary as we age – and the evidence shows it does – then lower-back pain becomes more likely. But moderate or vigorous activity also heightens the risk, whatever your age!

Tai chi has been shown to be effective in countering chronic pain (including the pain of osteoarthritis) and improving balance, strength in the lower limbs and general physical function, while countering fear of falling. Yoga is felt by many to be more effective than any other treatment for lower-back pain.

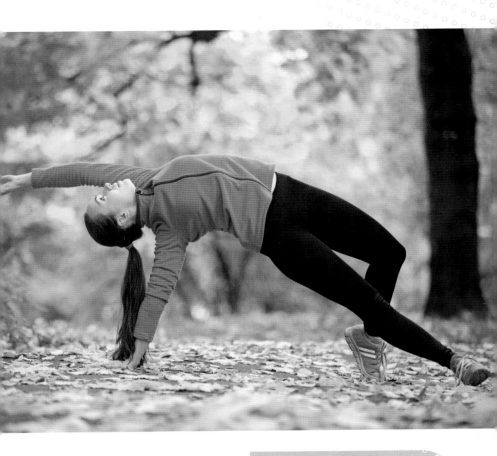

ABOVE: When the spine is able to move freely, the whole body can express itself with joy and spontaneity.

TIP: Stop smoking! It makes back pain more likely, by causing degenerative changes in the spine.

Seven star step

This is a beginner's pushing-hand drill that helps you explore the basic movements of tai chi. You take seven zigzagging steps forward and seven back, which helps to establish basic balance, coordination and transfer of bodyweight from side to side over the feet as well as building focus and concentration. Start slowly, building up to a more briskly zigzagging pace as the movements begin to feel more familiar.

1. Stand with feet hip-width apart, hands hanging loosely by your sides, looking forward.

2. Step diagonally forward with your left foot, following with the right foot. Your body faces diagonally to the left. Push your right palm out and bring your left hand up to the midline.

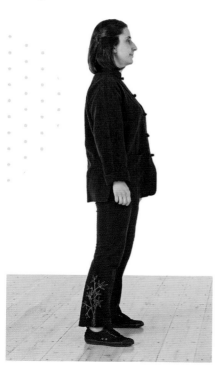
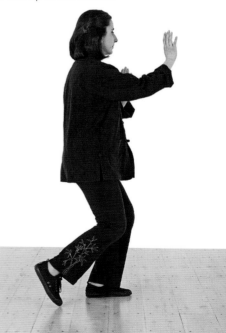

3. Now step diagonally forward with the right foot, letting the left foot follow. Your body faces diagonally to the right. Push your left palm forward and bring your right hand back to the midline.Repeat this stepping and pushing with alternate feet and hands a further five times.

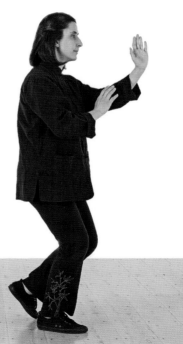

4. Then repeat the movement backward. Step back diagonally with your right foot, letting the left foot follow. Your body faces diagonally to the right. Push your left palm forward and draw your right hand back to the midline.

5. Step back diagonally with the left foot now, right foot following, as you turn your body to the left. Push your right palm forward and bring your left arm in, as before. Repeat the backward step and hand movements on alternate sides a further five times.

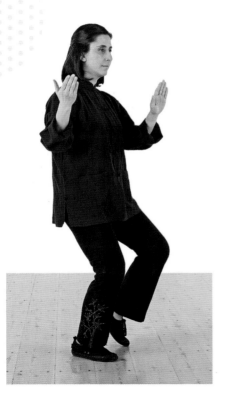
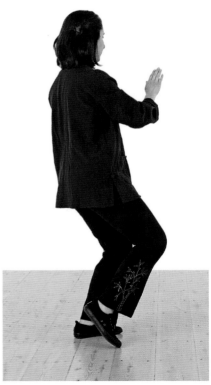

Yoga for healthy lower backs

One of the largest trials into yoga, conducted by the University of York, established that it was safe and effective for people with a history of lower-back pain. A 12-week programme of yoga led to greater improvement than did usual care. Here is a simple lower-back pain-relieving sequence based on the trial. Find the complete programme with a video to follow, plus details on where to take the 12-week course with a teacher, at http://www.yogaforbacks.co.uk

Rest position

The most important thing to do when you're in pain is to allow the body to find ease and the mind to become passive.

1. Start by lying on your back with a bolster or thick rolled blanket beneath the backs of your knees. Place a folded blanket beneath your head. If this feels too much, raise your lower legs, resting your calves on the seat of a chair, so the whole of your back rests on the floor and your lower legs are supported by the chair. This brings real relief and is helpful for pain in the sacroiliac joint between the sacrum and the pelvis.

2. Just rest here for 15 minutes. Cover yourself with a blanket if you tend to feel chilly when not moving.

3. Roll on to one side and push up to sitting or on to your hands and knees. You can either finish the exercise here, or move straight on to the exercises on pages 130–1.

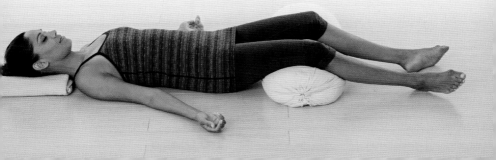

Table-top position

This hands-and-knees position can feel very stabilizing. Put a chair beneath your chest and rest your chest and stomach on the seat if that's more supportive.

1. Come on to all fours, with your hips over your knees and your hands a little in front of your shoulders. Hold for up to two minutes, rocking forward and back if that feels comfortable.

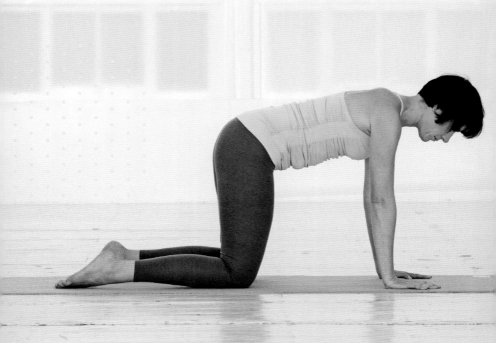

Lying twists

You don't need to take your legs to the ground in this exercise. You can hold the first step, or in the second step just take your knees an inch or so in either direction. If your back hurts, stop.

1. Lie on your back, with knees bent and feet hip-width apart. Relax here, feeling your back supported by the floor. Stay in this position if you like – you don't need to move on to the twists.

2. On an out-breath, take your knees very gently to the right, maybe only 1–2cm (about ½in). If that feels safe, take them halfway down, or if it's easy, bring them to rest on the floor. Turn your head to look at your left hand if that feels good.

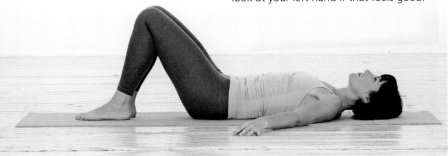

3. On an in-breath, bring the knees back up to centre. On another out-breath repeat to the other side.

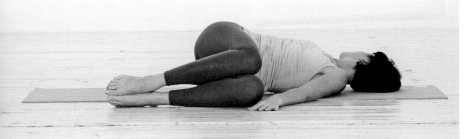

Upper-body strengthening

To free your spine from having to take the strain, don't neglect the muscles in the upper limbs, especially if you work the lower body a good deal with running or cycling. If you are able to support your bodyweight using your arms, wrists and hands, that keeps the back safe and switches on core muscles in the abdomen. Psychologically, it's uplifting to be able to do a press-up and hold it with your arms straight (Plank position).

Just as when the feet are active we can press into the floor to energize and activate the lower body, so when the hands and wrists are flexible and the arms strong we can press up from the floor to build strength in the upper body.

Arm and core strengthener

This yoga exercise uses your bodyweight as a training aid to build muscle in the arms and keep the wrists active. It makes a good build-up to the Plank and Chaturanga Poses, where you support your weight on your hands and toes (arms straight for Plank and bent for Chaturanga). It also builds core strength and tone in the pectoral muscles in the chest and supports the health and posture of the shoulders.

1. Start on all fours, hands beneath your shoulders and facing forward, knees beneath your hips. Then walk your hands forward by about 30cm (12in). Look slightly forward.

2. Push into your hands and use the upward force from the ground to pull your shoulder blades together and guide them down your back, toward your pelvis. Try to maintain that "set" position throughout the exercise.

3. As you exhale, pull your abdominal muscles back below your navel to support your spine. Maintain this tone and raise your right leg behind you. Notice whether you drop your abdominal tone or your arms wobble. If so, start again, focusing on keeping your lower back in the same position throughout.

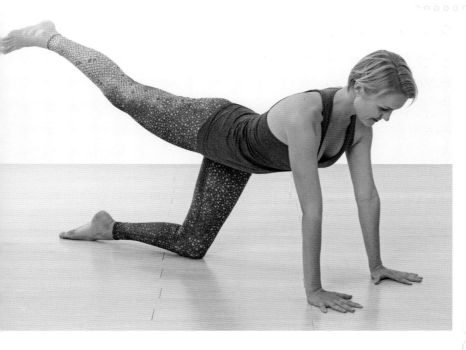

4. As you breathe out, bend your elbows, keeping them close to your waist and, looking forward, guide your chest toward the floor. You may descend just a tiny way; it's more important to keep your shoulder blades together, your navel lifted and elbows moving backward, not out to the side.

5. As you breathe in, push on your hands to straighten your arms. Check that your shoulders haven't rolled forward and your back is still protected – press back into your raised heel to prevent sagging. Repeat up to six times, maintaining good form – as soon as you start to sag, stop the exercise. Then repeat with the left leg extended.

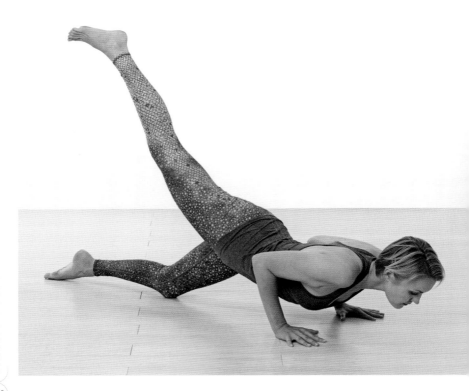

6. Once you've mastered the pose, you can try a full Chaturanga, starting with your legs outstretched in Plank pose and pressing back into your heels as you descend and hover just off the floor, before pushing back up.

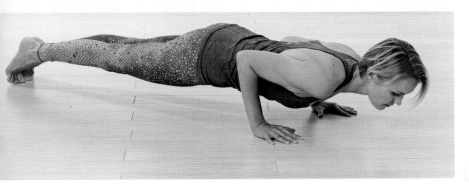

Forward punch

Another arm-strengthening exercise, this qigong sequence also builds stability in the lower back while working the arms and increasing good posture. Once you feel confident in the sequence, add free weights.

1. Start in horse stance, feet wider than hip-width apart and angled in line with your knees, and knees slightly bent. Sink your hips and lift your spine out of your pelvis. Have your hands at your waist, fists clenched and palms facing upward.

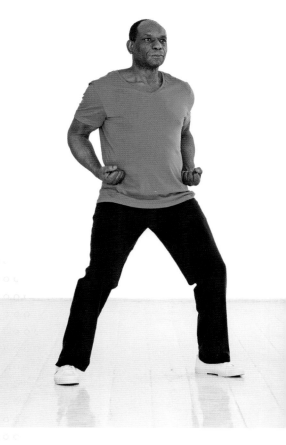

2. As you exhale, punch forward with your right wrist, turning it so the palm faces the floor when your arm is fully extended. Keep looking forward.

3. As you inhale, withdraw the fist, twisting it so that the palm faces upward again.

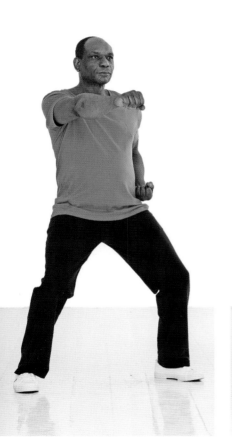

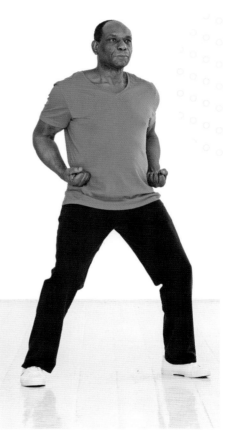

4. Now punch forward with your left fist on an exhalation, turning it again as you extend your arm so the palm faces down. Withdraw your left fist on the inhalation, twisting in the same way to return to the starting position. Repeat the sequence six times, alternating arms and keeping your attention focused forward and your posture strong and secure.

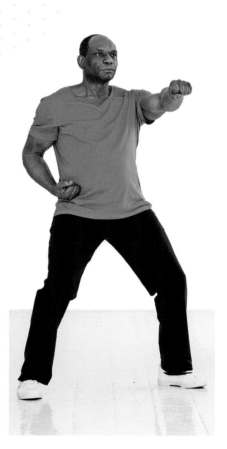
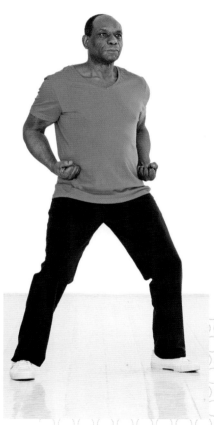

Wrist flexing

After taking pressure through the wrists in yoga poses, lifting weights or long periods at the computer, stretch out the arms to maximize flexibility and promote blood flow to the hands.

1. Sit or stand comfortably and stretch your arms out in front of you, palms facing down. Rotate at the wrists to circle your hands first in one direction for five circles, and then in the other direction for five. Don't move your arms, just your hands.

2. Now test your brain and coordination by seeing if you can rotate one wrist clockwise and one anticlockwise, then switch directions.

3. Press through the wrists so the palms face forward and fingers point up, holding for a count of five. Feel the stretch through the back of the arms.

4. Then drop the wrists, directing the fingers toward your forearms, again holding for five. Feel the stretch in the tops of the arms. Shake your arms and hands loosely to finish.

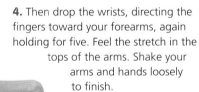

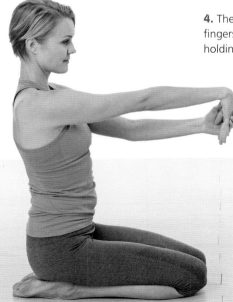

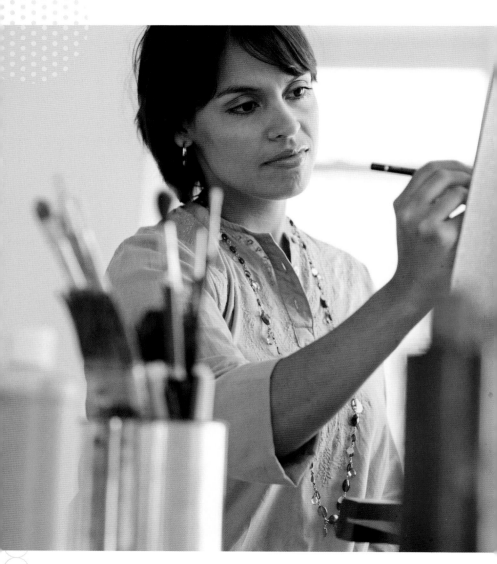

Rest and relaxation

Yes, we need to get more active in order to live longer and more satisfying lives, but the opposite of activity – rest – is as important in delaying the negative effects of ageing. It's part of the process of building strength and endurance, allowing the body systems restorative time to recuperate, rebuild and re-energize.

We need plenty of sleep (when growth hormone is produced to repair tissue and build muscle) and also plenty of "active rest" – not sitting on the sofa, but taking part in pleasurable pastimes that feel good for body and brain, such as walking the dog, swimming in the sea and being creative with paint, pen or music.

Lack of sleep has been studied in relation to cellular ageing, and some research suggests that lack of sleep is connected to shortened telomeres (these are found at the ends of our chromosomes – when they get too short, cells can no longer divide to repair the body; see page 14).

How do you know when you need more rest? Get into the habit of being mindful and noticing what's going on in your body. It's a good idea to keep a journal. Note down how well you slept, when you exercised, what you ate and how much rest you got. When did you decide to get the bus rather than walk home? At what point did your hip ache or cramps set in during an exercise session? You'll be able to spot patterns after a few weeks.

LEFT: Active rest is about making time for activities you love and that bring you into the present moment, such as absorbing creative pursuits.

Rest and training

If you want to stay fit into the later decades, ensure you weave the right amount of rest days into your workout schedule. If you train hard you need to rest the body properly on rest days, to make sure you're less likely to suffer injury or feel fatigued, stressed or moody.

Extreme sports need radical rest! Recovery days allow time for repair (of cognitive function, too) and are essential to being able to keep on moving like a younger body. Deep rest is especially supportive during the perimenopausal period, which can be marked by feelings of intense exhaustion. You may find you need to add in extra rest days, choose a restorative yoga class over an intense flow session or recast a weekly schedule over ten days or two weeks.

When to rest

Take a recovery day every third day when you're starting out on aerobic and endurance work, building up to one rest day a week. After two months of training most days, dial back for a week. If you're working the major muscle groups in your resistance training, leave a couple of days' rest before going back to the same area of the body, alternating a legs day with a back day and so on.

RIGHT: Yawning relaxes the jaw and diaphragm to allow deeper breathing and to prepare the body to rest well.

SIGNS YOU NEED A REST DAY

- Injury
- Constant stiffness or sore joints
- Colds or sickness
- Not achieving last week's times or weights
- You exercise regularly and your mind says you need a break

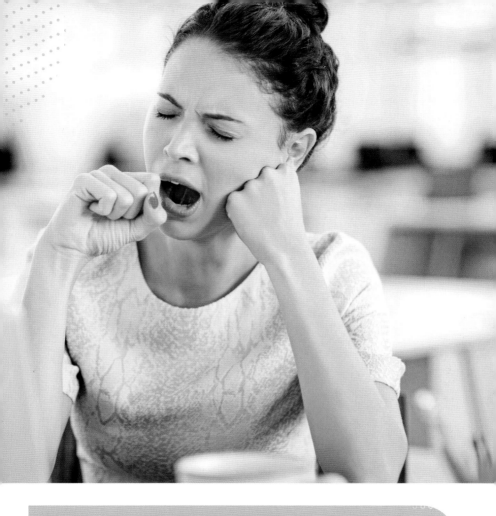

TIP: If talk of exercise makes you feel tired, you may need more exercise. Fatigue is thought to be as high as 50 per cent in older people, and research associates it with lower levels of physical activity, especially for women.

How much sleep?

Counter-intuitively, older adults need just as much sleep as younger adults – some seven to nine hours each night, and it's the same for men and women. That much sleep ensures we remain alert and well engaged during the day and allows adequate time at night for healing daily wear and tear to body and brain. Rapid eye movement (REM) dreaming sleep in particular, which makes up about a quarter of our night's sleep, is most restorative; that's when growth hormone is produced to repair and rebuild muscles and restore areas of the brain linked to learning, information storage and consolidating memory.

What does change with age is how we sleep. On the plus side, people over 55 tend to have a more consistent sleep routine (younger adults sleep less on week nights). But as we get older we can find it more difficult to drift off to sleep, women especially, and nights can be disturbed by periods of restlessness and waking.

During sleep, we move through 90-minute cycles made up of five different stages of sleep – two stages of light sleep, two of deep, slow-wave sleep and a short 15-minute burst of dreaming REM sleep – and the amount of time we spend in the various stages alters as we age. Older people tend to have longer light-sleep periods and less deep sleep.

INSOMNIA

This is more prevalent in older adults – according to a poll by the National Sleep Foundation, 44 per cent of older people in America experienced it for a few nights a week or more. Medical problems that have insomnia as a side-effect are also more prevalent. These include high blood pressure, respiratory and immune disorders, and menopausal symptoms such as night sweats. Not sleeping well as we age can make our quality of life feel worse and feed a number of health problems, including depression, reduced attention span and memory lapses, and increased use of medication. It's also linked to increased falls at night. In MRI scans of people who haven't slept, there is much less activity in the areas of the brain used in decision-making, memory recall and problem-solving. If you feel lack of sleep is reducing your quality of life or contributing to health problems, consult a doctor or sleep specialist.

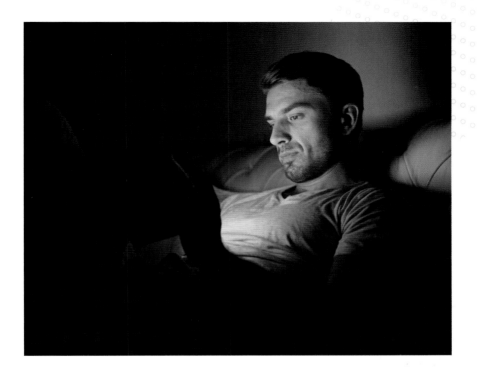

In light sleep we're easily disturbed by environmental factors, such as noise or heat, or internal stimuli, such as restless legs. Once awake, it's harder to segue to the next stage of sleep.

We may have the urge to go to bed earlier in the evening as we age, or find we wake earlier. If you're used to sleeping in or have previously been a night owl, this can be disconcerting, even if you're still getting your seven to nine hours. Napping during the day is more common

ABOVE: Dim your screen before bed – use an app that decreases blue light or read white type on a black background – and choose passive activities such as reading.

TIP: If you feel restless in bed, try an extra blanket tucked in firmly or a compression quilt. As with swaddling a baby, gentle but firm pressure that stops the limbs from jerking can calm the nervous system and feel very comforting.

with age, especially after a disturbed night. It's not a good idea to fall asleep on the sofa in the early evening because that prevents us from moving neatly on to the next stage of sleep once in bed.

Why might sleep patterns change with age? It's not well understood, but reduced secretion of melatonin might contribute. Melatonin is the hormone produced by the pineal gland that regulates our sleep/wake patterns – when the light level drops, melatonin is released, which triggers the body systems to slow down.

The other thing that's changed as the years have passed – regardless of how old we are – is our use of screens. The blue light emitted by LED backlit screens and monitors suppresses the release of melatonin, and a decline in sleep duration in industrialized countries has been linked with the rise in screen time. However, the problem may be more a question of what you do with the screen. Research by the US National Sleep Foundation shows that people who watched a film slept more easily than those who were interactive, playing games, answering emails or texting. The latter were more stressed and had poorer sleep.

THE ABC OF NAPPING

The ability to nap during the day may be worth cultivating as we age – it seems to correlate with enhanced cognitive performance. In research on people between the ages of 50 and 83, napping – whether for 45 minutes or two hours – didn't seem to impact on either the quality or duration of night-time sleep, but did contribute significantly to the total amount of sleep participants got over 24 hours. Surveys of almost 3,000 older Chinese people found that those who took a post-lunch snooze of about an hour had better recall, memory and ability to stay attentive. Napping may also lower blood pressure. But what makes a good nap as we age?

• Longer seems more effective than shorter – aim for nearer an hour than 20 minutes.

• Make it a habit – build it into your day, maybe after lunch.

• Don't take a nap too late in the day; doing so may affect your night-time sleep cycle.

• If you feel tired but can't nap, take a short walk instead – it's as effective in refreshing the brain.

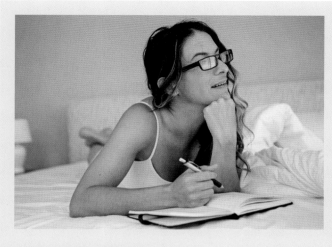

LEFT: Keeping a journal for morning thoughts on waking and downloading lists or worries before bed frees the mind for restful sleep.

GOOD SLEEP ESSENTIALS

• Exercise most days, ideally in the morning.

• Be sociable during the day.

• Eat sleep-enhancing foods (oats, bananas, almonds, turkey, lettuce) and avoid caffeine from the afternoon onward.

• Spend time outdoors to maximize the production of serotonin (a neurotransmitter that helps to regulate mood and encourage sleep).

• Keep the bedroom clean, well aired and free from work and technology.

• Reserve the bed for sex and sleep.

• Set up a bedtime routine.

• If you spend long periods of the night awake, go to bed late and get up early.

• Don't measure sleep by hours but by how you feel.

• Keep a record of your sleep habits, if you need a better fix on what's real and what you're imagining.

Healthy bedtime routine

In a study of over-65s by the National Institute on Aging, 36 per cent of women (and 13 per cent of men) found it took longer than 30 minutes to drop off. A regular pre-bed routine was found to be effective in teaching body and mind to switch into an off state that made deep sleep more likely.

Oiling the body

Massage with a soporific oil before bed is a good way to start the wind-down process. In the Ayurvedic text the *Ashtanga Hridayam*, oiling the body daily (*abhyanga*) is said to reverse and prevent ageing while increasing longevity. The traditional application is of sweet almond, mustard or sesame oil, rubbed into the spine, head and feet. The circular massaging movements stimulate the lymphatic and immune systems, carrying nutrients to, and waste away from, cells while calming and balancing the nervous and hormonal systems. The oils can be blended with two drops of essential oil of lavender, or with herbs and essential oils that rebalance your Ayurvedic constitution (see page 17).

The oil should be applied a couple of hours after eating (warm it in winter by standing the bottle in a mug of warm water). It's more relaxing if someone else does the applying, but you could treat your feet, legs, arms and even your head yourself. Strokes are not considered too important in Ayurvedic massage – it's more about feeding the skin. Work progresses upward from the soles of the feet, with most time spent on the feet and head. A stronger pressure can be applied in these places. Work on the back and around the spine should be done very carefully and gently. Rest in Corpse Pose (*Savasana*, see page 154) after being massaged, and leave the oil on the skin for at least an hour to be absorbed before bathing or showering. Some people like to visit a sauna afterward. Oiling the scalp is said to be restorative for hair loss.

BUILD AN EFFECTIVE SLEEP ROUTINE

• Set yourself a regular bedtime (before midnight) and regular waking time and make every effort to stick to it.

• Disengage from technology by instigating an "electronic sunset" at least an hour before bed.

• If you're a worrier, create a paper list journal and fill it in before bed; doodle and colour if that feels good, or try the Box Visualization (see page 152).

• Create darkness with blackout blinds if it's not dark outside.

• Drink warm milk sweetened with two teaspoons of honey. Honey is thought to be the best food for storing glycogen in the liver. The glycogen fuels the brain overnight and prevents the release of stress hormones (also good for prolonged periods of exertion or exercise).

• Keep the sensory stimulus low as you go to bed – a quiet, well-aired room, smooth sheets and dimmed lights mean less sleep disturbance.

• Put two drops of essential oil of lavender in a diffuser or bowl of hot water and leave in the bedroom for 30 minutes before bed. In a study, people who did this were better able to reach a state of deep sleep and awoke more refreshed next morning. Or add to a massage blend (see opposite).

• Relax in silence in a bath or with bedtime reading or guided meditation.

• Practise yoga poses such as Inverted Pose (*Viparita Karani*, see page 342) or Supported Child's Pose (*Adhomukha Virasana*, see page 153) or try the yoga breathing practices on pages 292–3.

• Use a deep-relaxation technique such as Yoga Nidra (see page 154).

• Keep a glass of water by your bedside.

Queen of the night

The great goddess comprises three "aspects" or times of life: maiden, mother and crone. In the Greek pantheon, the crone is Hecate. Her time is the waning and dark moon, and although her power extends over earth, sea and heavens, it is with the other world and darkness that she is most often associated. She can pass into the underworld but doesn't dwell there, instead inhabiting a cave between our world and the next. Her place is the twilight between states, a liminal zone between this world and unknowable futures. This mysterious moon goddess is often depicted with three heads, or as three figures facing in different directions, for she is mistress of the crossroads, able to see three ways at once: past, present and future. Her long life has equipped her with wisdom and intuition. This makes her a useful aid to contemplation at times of transition, when there are midlife choices to be made, or in the small hours when menopause-disturbed sleep assaults us with questions and searching, regrets and possibilities.

Although Hecate is associated with darkness, thanks to her there is regeneration. It is she who, with energy and persistence, seeks out and uncovers the truth, counsels in times of loss, and with flaming torches and a headband of stars guides Demeter on through the dark of the night to find her lost child, Persephone. Without Persephone, there can be no spring each year, and Hecate henceforth is Persephone's invisible companion. Without sleep there is no renewal, without the barrenness of winter no eventual new shoots of life.

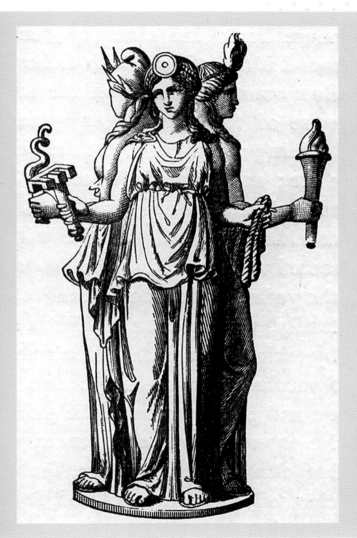

LEFT: The goddess Hecate in her triple form depicted with a key with which to open gates, a flaming torch to light the underworld, and a serpent, symbol of healing as well as death.

Box visualization

This is a useful way to put aside worries before bed.
Sit or lie comfortably with your eyes closed.

1. Imagine you have a beautiful wooden box with a lid. Look at the outside; perhaps it's intricately carved or painted with reassuring symbols and patterns that mean something to you. In your mind's eye see the thickness of the sides, the way the lid fits snugly on top. Look inside at the soft lining. Perhaps it's velvet, the softest cotton wool or feathery down.

2. Think about what's concerning you and put a symbol of it in the box for safe-keeping while you sleep. It could be a pair of baby shoes, the keys to a house, a memory stick or a photograph of someone.

3. Now put the box somewhere safe where you can't see it – in a cave, in the middle of a huge field or on a high shelf in a cupboard. Walk away from the box, letting go of the thoughts about what's inside because you know that the box is there quite safe, waiting for you to return to it tomorrow.

Supported child's pose *(Adhomukha Virasana)*

Forward bends help to close down the front of the body (where the sense organs sit) and calm the nervous system. The props in this pose support the sternum and put a little pressure on the forehead, which is intensely calming.

1. Sit on your heels with your knees wide. Place a bolster lengthways in front of you and a rolled blanket horizontally across the end, to make a T-shape. With your toes touching, slowly fold forward, laying your abdomen and then your chest on the bolster. Rest your forehead on the blanket. Adjust the props until you feel completely peaceful. You can stretch your arms in front of you or bring them to rest beside your body, hands next to your feet.

2. Rest in this position for up to five minutes (or ten if you find it relaxing). Notice the in-breath filling and expanding the back of your body – diverting attention from the sense organs in the front of the body can be a relief.

3. To come up, stretch your hands forward and press through your palms to push yourself up, bringing your head up last.

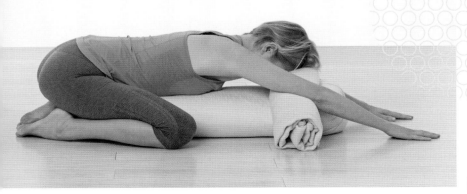

Supported corpse pose *(Savasana)* with guided yoga nidra

This supported relaxation position promotes deep rest and allows your energy to gather in from the peripheries. You'll need three folded blankets, a rolled towel and a bolster. In the pose we'll practise Yoga Nidra, or deep yoga sleep. Set aside a good 15–30 minutes to benefit from the practice.

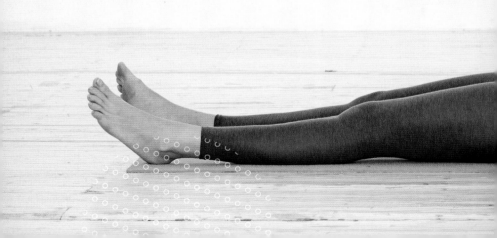

1. Lie on your back (in bed is fine or supported with blankets and bolsters). Relax your arms away from your body, palms facing upward, and stretch your legs away comfortably, feet flopping outward. Make sure you feel warm and well supported.

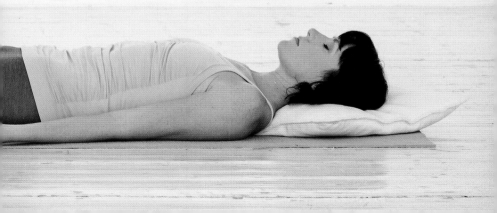

2. If you don't feel relaxed, have a wriggle and adjust until you feel able to settle. Now sink into the stillness, feeling the ground or bed supporting your pelvis and head, shoulders and heels.

3. Watch your breath moving in and out. Don't try to alter it, just be aware of how it is. Then on the out-breaths allow everything to drop into the support beneath you. Know you are held here safely. Say to yourself, "I am practising Yoga Nidra." If you'd like to add a resolve – to sleep more soundly, to feel calmer – do that and then let it go.

4. You're going to guide your awareness around your body as it rests on the floor. Imagine it as a tiny torchlight picking out each part of your body in turn; or you might like to picture the tip of a magic wand or soft feather lightly brushing each body part. Take your inner gaze to the back of your head, your right ear lobe, the right side of your jaw, your left ear lobe and jaw, your teeth, your top teeth, your bottom teeth, your tongue, your

lips. Take the light to your right eye, your left eye, your forehead, your eyebrows and eyelashes top and bottom, your cheekbones, your cheeks. Be aware of your whole head.

5. Move down your neck now to your right shoulder, armpit, upper arm, elbow, inner elbow, lower arm, wrist, palm and all the fingers. Linger as you shine the light on each one in turn. Be aware of the right side of your body. Now move down your left side from neck to fingertips in the same way.

6. Travel down your torso, shining your light on your chest, between each rib front and back, down your breastbone, your upper abdomen, around the navel, lower abdomen, the bones of the pelvis, the tailbone. Be aware of your torso.

7. Guide your mind's eye down your right thigh, knee, back of knee, calf, ankle. Follow down the front of the foot, heel of the foot, arch of the foot, down to the big toe and all the toes to the little toe.

Be aware of your whole right leg. Follow the same pattern down the left leg and foot, and be aware of your whole left leg.

8. Observe your whole body in the deeply relaxed state of Yoga Nidra. Feel the back of the body heavy on the floor but the front of the body light and free, able to breathe easily. Enjoy the dark space between the eyes. Return to your intention if you set one.

9. Become aware of your breathing now. Become aware of your body in space and of the room around you. Notice any sounds or sensations. Lie for a while just noticing; no need to think or do anything. When you feel ready, gently move your fingers and toes and the tip of your tongue. Roll onto one side and rest here before moving or falling asleep.

WHAT IS YOGA NIDRA?

This method of intense body relaxation relaxes the physical body but also works on the mind and emotions to release tension and bring about a transformative state of awareness akin to self-hypnosis. It feels incredibly nourishing and replenishing, and hypnotherapy seems to be a good tool for improving sleep affected by the menopause.

Yoga Nidra is best led by an experienced teacher, although after experiencing it you can replicate some of the experience yourself, with practice guiding yourself through the process more intuitively. There are very good Yogra Nidra podcasts available from the inspirational teacher Uma Dinsmore-Tuli and others here: yoganidranetwork.org/ downloads

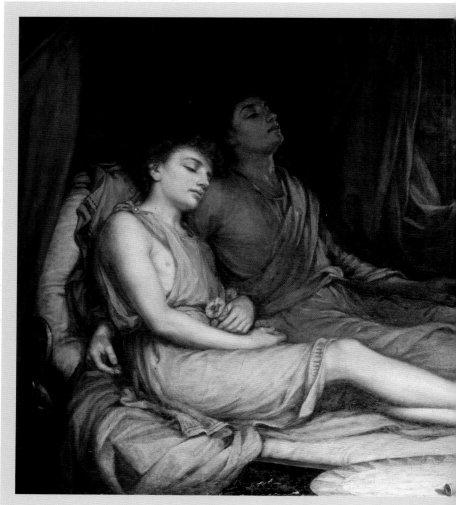

ABOVE: Sleep and his brother Death, as envisaged by the artist John William Waterhouse in 1874.

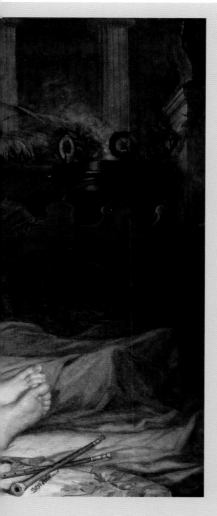

Kind sleep

In the Greek pantheon, sleep is Hypnos, brother to Death (Thanatos), and they are children of Night. Sleep is the benevolent sibling. Gentlest of the gods, he "roams peacefully over the earth and the sea's broad back and is kindly to men," Hesiod tells us. He brings sleep by touching mortals very gently with his magic wand or with a brush of his soft dark wings. So effective is his power that he can bring even the greatest of the gods to a state of slumber – Hera asks him to take the form of a night bird to lull Zeus, king of the gods, to sleep. Night's home is a dark and "dumb quiet" cave at the place where night and day meet. It's filled with the seed heads of poppies that bloom in abundance nearby, and Lethe, the river of forgetfulness, has its source here, bubbling up and trickling over little pebbles. As we sleep, Hypnos sends out his son Morpheus – Ovid's "mastercraftsman and simulator of human forms" – the winged messenger who delivers and shapes our dreams.

Toning and relaxing the face

The loss in muscle strength and elasticity we experience throughout the body as we age is perhaps most evident in the facial muscles and the texture of the complexion. Signs of ageing in men are gradual. In women, they rise markedly from our 40s as our hormones change – in our early 30s we look younger than men because our monthly hormones keep the skin soft.

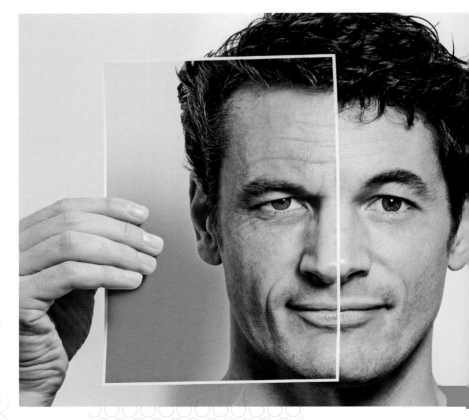

Declining muscle tone affects the upper eyelids in particular, and is also seen in a softening of tone around the nose and chin, ears and lips. Ligaments around the nose, mouth and chin relax, causing these features to droop, while cartilage in the ears becomes lax and adds to elongation.

In some parts of the face we build stronger muscles with age – through habitual frowning or scowling, which shows in particular between the brows and across the forehead. The more often and more forcefully we react in this way to the world, the more the lines become etched in and remain, even in repose.

We lose subcutaneous fat from the face through the decades, and fat stores shift in position; without this underpinning volume, skin begins to loosen and fold and becomes more susceptible to gravity, dropping downward especially around the cheeks and jawline. Fat helps support the eyes and cheeks, so when it starts to decline, and the tissue thins, these features can sink, while others, such as the brow ridges, seem more prominent. Thinning of the dermis layer brings a look of transparency, while declining production of elastin (which allows skin to return to shape) and collagen (governing stretch and strength) add to the ageing effect.

Exercising the facial muscles can help mitigate the effects, and as with all exercise, it's important to balance toning with relaxation, and learn to let go of the habitual ways in which we hold tension in the face. But you need to do more than work on the facial muscles in order to relax the face – releasing tension in the feet with a massage (see page 82) or foot exercises can have a remarkably

LEFT: The trick with good ageing is to love the age you're becoming and to acknowledge the changes rather than hide behind a mask.

rejuvenating effect on the way we hold our features.

Relaxation of the facial muscles starts with mindfulness, being aware of our habits and response patterns (and trying to be non-judgmental). Do you find yourself scowling or grimacing as you work? Clenching your jaw or frowning as you concentrate? Stooping forward as you text or holding the phone between shoulder and ear? That tension can settle into the face. The eye area suffers in particular from techno-overload when we spend long hours at screens; exercising the eyes releases tension in the face as well as helping with dizziness and fear of falling.

Facial yoga is especially useful in retraining us to soften and relax habitual patterns of holding that make us look strained. It also encourages us to think kindly about how we look as the years pass, and to find ways to continue presenting ourselves with confidence to the world.

INSTANT FACIAL FIX

To relax the face, close your eyes and imagine the space between your eyebrows widening. Feel your forehead smoothing out and the sides of your eyes growing out into your temples. Relax your jaw and feel more space in your mouth.

SKIN PROTECTION FROM THE OUTSIDE

The main cause of skin ageing – from wrinkles to age spots – is ultraviolet (UV) damage caused by exposure to the sun. Choose factor-50 sunscreens for face and hands, and look for products that protect against ultraviolet A (UVA) as well as ultraviolet B (UVB) light. (UVA is most ageing for the skin – look for products with four or five stars for good protection). Studies show that we don't apply enough sunscreen, so put more on your face and neck than you think you need, about a teaspoonful, and replenish every couple of hours. Moisturizers and foundations, concealers and powder-finish formulations that contain a sunscreen are good for layering.

RIGHT: Releasing tension held in the neck and shoulders can have a relaxing and rejuvenating effect on the muscles of the face.

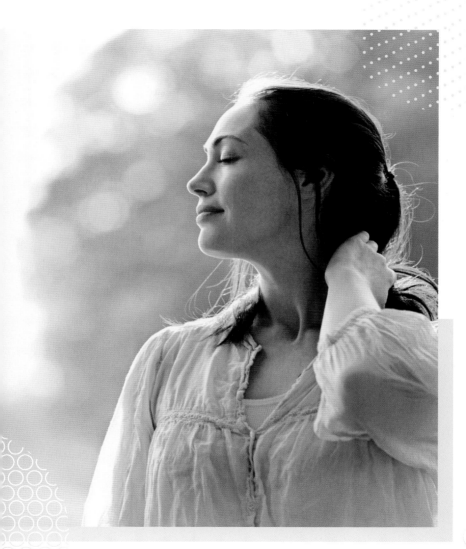

Start with the shoulders

We absorb a good deal of tension in the neck and shoulders, so releasing the shoulders is the first step in easing a tense face. This blissful release also stretches the backs of the legs and feels good on the back. Try it after a period of sitting at a computer. Cushion your elbows with a folded blanket if they feel uncomfortable on the hard surface.

1. Stand half a body's length from a table or flat support. Either have your feet hip-width apart or keep your right foot facing forward and take a good step back with your left foot, angling it out slightly.

2. Bend your knees and bow forward carefully to rest your elbows and upper arms on the table, shoulder-width apart. Shuffle until your arms and legs feel comfortable, your head is in line with your spine and there's a good stretch in your upper arms and shoulders.

3. Bring your palms to touch above your head. Hold the position, breathing smoothly for 30 seconds or longer, feeling the stretch all the way along your spine.

4. Once you've settled in the pose, try bringing your palms onto your upper back – this increases the stretch for some people and eases it for others. Straighten your legs if that feels good, bringing your hips in line (move your right hip back). Come up slowly on an inhalation and repeat on the other side if you practised with legs apart.

Neck release

After stretching the shoulders, release the muscles that hold up the head and align the neck. This sequence helps to pinpoint the stretch your neck needs (we all hold tension in a slightly different area).

1. Sit or kneel in a comfortable position, resting your hands in your lap. Close your eyes and tune in to your breathing. Feel your spine rising tall out of your pelvis and a pull upward at the crown of your head.

2. Place one palm on your forehead, with the heel of your hand resting at the third-eye area (see page 339). Exhale and press your forehead against your palm to set up a resistance for a count of three or four. Keep your chin tucked in slightly. Inhale and release the pressure. Repeat with the other palm.

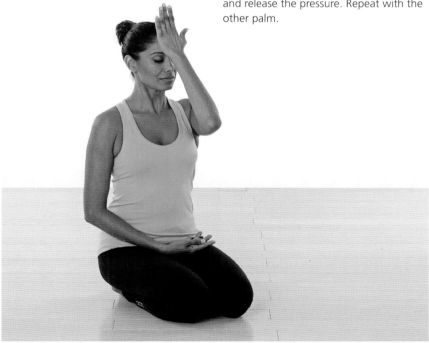

3. Interlace your fingers and cup the back of your head in your palms. With your chin tucked in slightly, exhale and press your head back into your palms for a count of three or four. Inhale, release your arms, interlink your fingers the other way (with the non-habitual index finger on top) and repeat.

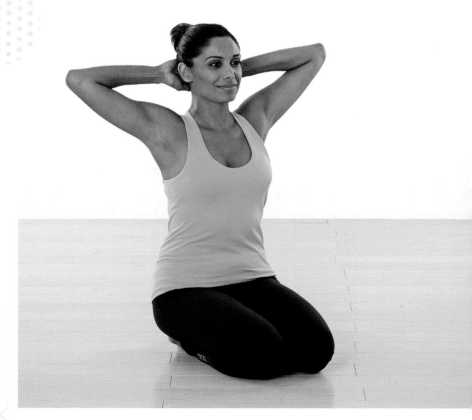

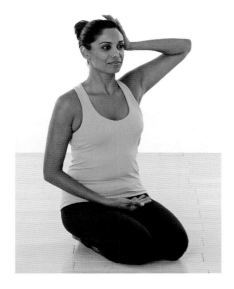

4. Place your palm on the side of your head now, against your ear, and exhaling, press the side of your head into your palm for a count of three or four. Inhale and release. Repeat, then do the same on the other side of your head.

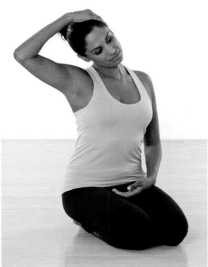

5. Finally, tilt your right ear toward your right shoulder, feeling a stretch down the left side of your neck. Drop your left shoulder. This may give you enough stretch. If not, reach your right arm over your head and rest the palm of your hand on the side of your head to add very gentle pressure. Exhale and resist the pressure with your head for a count of three or four and then release. Inhale to release your arm and bring your head back to centre. Repeat on the other side.

Facial qigong

Use these exercises to work the muscles around the mouth, cheek, jaw and eye area. Try not to crease up other areas of the face as you concentrate on the muscle-strengthening.

1. Bring your teeth together, then slowly smile widely with your lips open, stretching the sides of the mouth toward your ears as if saying "eee". Really stretch the lower lip. Hold the position while tapping your teeth together lightly and slowly 36 times. This exercises the muscles of the lower third of the face, including strengthening the lower cheek, neck and sides of the mouth. The tapping relaxes the jaw. Move the corners of your mouth back in very slowly.

2. Bring your lips together and very slowly widen the sides of the mouth again, teeth together. Then raise your chin. Swallow three times before lowering the chin and releasing the mouth position slowly. This exercises the muscles of the neck and jawline. In Traditional Chinese Medicine swallowing saliva is said to aid digestion and longevity.

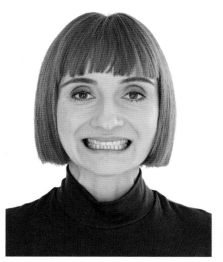
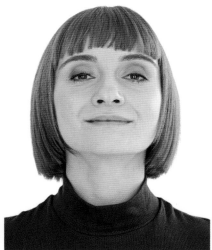

3. To strengthen the upper eyelid muscles, place your middle fingers on your eyebrows, one on each side. Hold the skin beneath the eyebrows firmly, anchoring it to the bone, then slowly close your eyes by dropping your eyelids over your eyes; feel a tension from brow to lashes. Hold the eyes shut for a count of five, then release as slowly as you closed them. Repeat three times.

4. To encourage the brow muscles to release tension, place your fingers between your eyebrows and pull out toward your temples, keeping the skin taut. Rest your fingertips at your temples for a moment before repeating three times. As you draw your fingers away from your temples try to maintain the sense of a smooth brow.

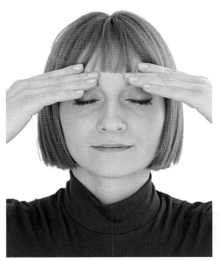
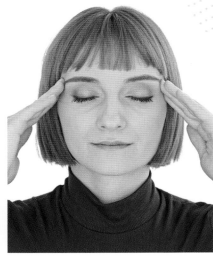

Eye exercises

Yoga eye exercises not only work the muscles around the eye area, they help us isolate movement in one part of the body – being able to focus on and move a single area increases mental agility. Blink between exercises to moisten the eyes – one in three people over 65 reportedly has problems with dry eyes and we blink less often when using a screen. Dry-eye syndrome is linked with the hormonal changes of menopause.

1. Sit or kneel in a comfortable position, resting your hands in your lap. Close your eyes and tune in to your breathing. Keep your face still, relax your neck and shoulders and make the following movements with your eyes only.

2. Look up and hold for five. Look down and hold for five. Then return your gaze to the centre.

3. Look to the right and hold for five. Check you haven't moved your chin. Slide your eyes to the left and hold, then return your gaze to centre.

4. Now look top right and bottom left. Look top left and bottom right. Return your gaze to centre, then close and rest your eyes.

5. Look at something close to you; focus on it without straining. Now find an object in the distance and fix your gaze on it. Finally, blur your gaze by widening your eyes and unfocusing slightly, as if looking out through your temples. Close your eyes and rest.

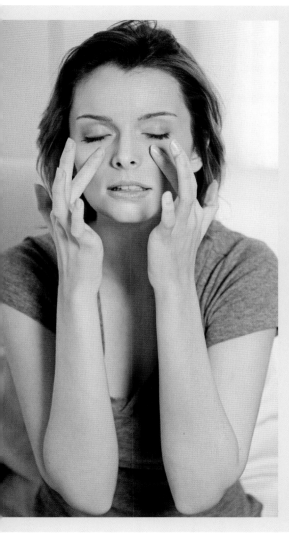

FACIAL MASSAGE OIL

Choose rosehip oil (*Rosa mosqueta*) for facial massage twice a day. Thanks to its essential fatty acids, this oil has skin-repair properties, reducing visible signs of sun damage and hyper-pigmentation as well as scar tissue. Essential oil of rose (*Rosa centifolia* or *R. damascena*) is valued by aromatherapists and added to massage-oil blends for bringing balance to perimenopausal symptoms, quelling anxiety and easing the effects of stress while encouraging rest and deepening feelings of femininity and sexuality. It is also added to oil blends for restoring sensitive, inflamed or ageing skin.

LEFT: Use the middle fingers to massage around the eyes, for the lightest pressure and most delicate touch.

Downward-facing dog pose *(Adhomukha Svanasana)*

You can't beat this yoga pose for its anti-gravity effect on the face and neck. It has all the benefits of an inversion, pumping freshly oxygenated blood to the face to boost the complexion. It's an all-star pose, building strength in the hands, wrists and arms while lengthening the muscles along the back of the body. Avoid inversions if you have high blood pressure, glaucoma or a detached retina.

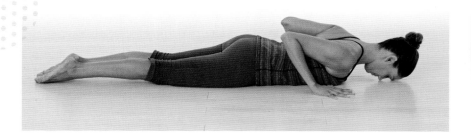

1. Lie on your front with your legs outstretched and forehead on the floor. Place your hands beneath your shoulders, elbows tucked in. This helps find the most effective stretch position for your body.

2. Push into your hands to lift into an all-fours position, toes tucked under and feet hip-width apart. Roll your inner thighs back and your lower spine in.

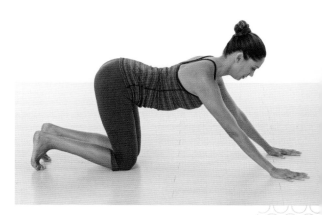

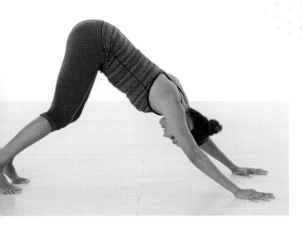

3. Keep pushing on your palms to take your bottom back and up. Rise high onto tiptoes and keep your knees bent. It's more important to get your bottom high and your back straight than to straighten your legs. Stop here if this is enough.

4. Take your thighs back and guide your heels toward the floor – it's not important that they get there. Check your hands are facing forward and all your fingers are working hard. Press into the base of your index fingers and thumbs and stretch away from that point. Enjoy the lovely stretch up your arms and back and down your legs. Visualize the blood flowing to your face to energize and plump up the skin.

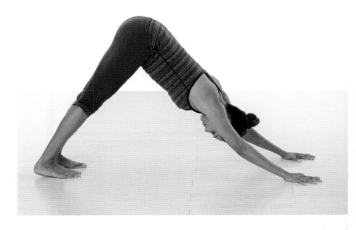

Facial relaxation

This total body relaxation with a softening visualization helps to release long-held tension in the face. With the head and neck supported on pillows, it also encourages gravity to drain away any puffiness. You will need bolsters and a blanket.

1. Set up for relaxation by placing the bolster vertically with the folded blanket toward the top. Sit in front of the bolster and relax back onto it, so your head and neck are raised by the blanket, your back is well supported on the bolster and there's a good opening through your chest. Shuffle forward if the end of the bolster isn't comfortable in your lower back. Relax your hands on the floor away from your body, palms facing up.

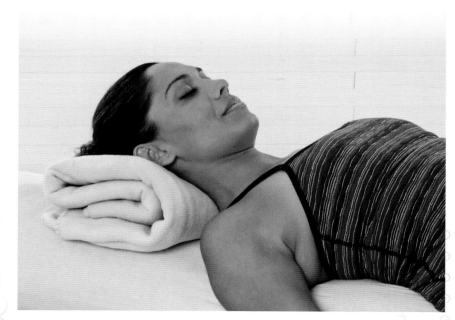

2. Close your eyes and watch your breath moving in and out for a few breaths. Imagine the skin on your face, scalp and neck softening and draping beautifully over your bones. Rest here for five to ten minutes, letting go of tension in each of the following in turn: your jaw, your ears, the back of your head, the hair follicles, your forehead, your eyes, your eyelids, your eyebrows, your lips, your tongue, the pores of your skin. Let your mouth be soft, your tongue relaxed, tip resting behind your teeth, lips slightly parted with a soft smile. Feel your eyes heavy in the sockets and the lids perfectly smooth over them. Focus at the third eye (see page 339) if that feels comfortable. Visualize gravity smoothing the skin on your forehead toward your temples. When you notice tension or a twitch, consciously relax it, then stop thinking and allow yourself to drift off.

RELAXATION SCENTS

Add a few drops of the following essential oils to a diffuser to encourage relaxation. These are considered very feminine scents, good for the skin and traditionally used to support women during stressful times of transition or loss. Note: always buy essential oils from a reputable supplier.

- **Melissa:** for restful sleep, to ease anxiety and menopausal symptoms.
- **Jasmine:** for its uplifting and aphrodisiac qualities.
- **Geranium:** to rebalance the nervous system and for menopausal symptoms.
- **Bergamot:** to lift the spirits and enhance mood if you're feeling over-emotional.
- **Rose:** to relieve sadness, for menopausal symptoms and to encourage contemplation.

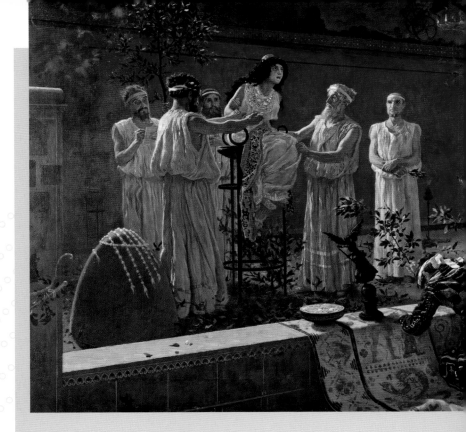

Wisdom of the hag

We fetishize young skin and have a fear, and often very visceral loathing, of ageing skin – its wrinkles, its dryness, the sagging – especially on women. In folklore, the witch shares the magical powers of the fairy – to grant wishes, to transform, to curse – but she's feared and despised, not welcomed to the party. She's depicted as an old wrinkled woman whose face is fearful to look

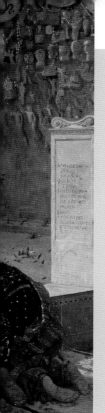

upon – a hag. "Repulsive old woman" with a "hideously malformed face" is the dictionary definition. The term is always used pejoratively. The word "hag" may derive from an old English word for hedge or boundary, *haga*, suggesting that she's someone on the edge, an outsider positioned at the limits of civilization where society blurs into wildness.

As our faces start to age we can feel similarly shunned, edged out, not part of the mainstream, but there's hope in the hag! Feminist folklorists have sought to reclaim her, pointing out that the word "hag" may share a root with the Greek *hagia*, or holy. Think of the Hagia Sophia church in Istanbul, built to honour the holy wisdom of Our Lady (*sophia* means wisdom). The word "hag" was certainly used to translate the names of prophetic women with supernatural powers in Greek tales, such as the harpies, the Furies and the voice of the Oracle at Delphi. The hag's wisdom – her ability to prophesy, heal and soothsay – comes from a life long-lived and lessons learned from hard-won experience. Mainstream society can feel threatened by outsiders with such power; it's safest to keep them at the edge. We might choose to align ourselves with the fearsome power of the outsider as we age. Then we can love our wrinkles not only as a sign of how much wisdom we have, but as a way to fight the powers that be.

Abkhazia, where beauty means age

Bounded by Georgia to the south and Russia to the north lies the independent republic of Abkhazia, feted for the age to which its inhabitants live – reputed 150th, 161st and 168th birthdays are written about and photographed. Anthropologist Sula Benet claimed in a 1970s study of the region that the Abkhaz had no word for "old people", and that it was age that denoted beauty, status and privilege here, rather than wealth or youth.

The picture was popularized in the 1970s by Harvard scientist Dr Alexander Leaf and a *National Geographic* photographer, who sought to track down and study the most long-lived communities around the globe. Dr Leaf wanted to analyse the lifestyle and beliefs of centenarians who maintained an active healthy life, to examine their blood pressure and pulse, vision and hearing. In Abkhazia, he tracked elderly men bounding up and down mountains and bathing vigorously in ice-cold water (Abkhazia lies between the Black Sea coast and the Caucasus mountains). He watched them sing in choirs where every member was over 100.

It's likely that the traditional way of life in this crescent of mountain and coast contributes to a healthy life – plenty of daily physical activity (these are mountain people, like many Dr Leaf studied), a diet rich in vegetables, fruit and fermented milk, with wine and moderate amounts of protein but little fat or carbohydrates (Dr Leaf found that 70 per cent of calories here came from vegetables), plus periods of fasting-like calorie restriction, all associated with longevity. Older people were valued for passing on the traditional way of life and culture and they played a key role in close but extended families while continuing to work into their later decades – more traits associated with longevity.

However, that's not the whole story. The people studied were born before births were recorded, when literacy was rare. And the Soviet regime approved and publicized the mythology of life spans longer than those of contemporary Americans.

If these elders were superfit and active, it may be down to genes. Until the 1860s the region was isolated for millennia and the language is unrelated to others in the region (said to be the hardest-sounding in the world, with 60 consonants to just one to four vowels). In the 1860s the Tsarist regime deported people to Turkey and ethnic Russians and Georgians moved in. Since then the state has been fought over, invaded and blockaded, borders closed and towns besieged. The war in the 1990s against Georgia caused the demographic to change again, as Georgians fled and the population halved. War and longevity don't mix.

Longevity still has a pull for outsiders here, though. Russians head to Abkhazia to take advantage of its mineral-water healing and grape cures. Then there's the unique geography – Mediterranean meets sub-tropical, with figs and pomegranates growing beside palms, and warm seas washing up to forested mountains with snow-capped peaks – a promising place to search for the secret of a long and beautiful life.

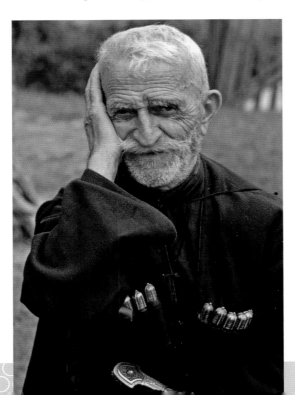

LEFT: An elderly, but youthful, Abkhazian man wears traditional dress from the region.

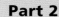

Part 2

LONGEVITY FOOD:
plants, variety, slowness

To add healthy years to our lives, as well as masses of
exercise we need really good nutrition in order to protect
the heart and cognitive function, maximize the health of
bones and joints, and lower the risks of getting a chronic
disease — according to the World Health Organization, all the
degenerative diseases of older age are affected by diet.

Although the principles of eating healthily are the same regardless of age – namely that people who eat plenty of plant foods are less likely to develop life-limiting heart disease and some cancers – nutritional requirements do change over the decades. We tend to be less physically active after the age of 40, our lean body mass decreases and body fat increases, and with the added reduction in hormones the metabolism starts slowing. Our need for energy follows suit. Put simply, we need to eat a bit less after the age of 50 for women and 60 for men.

If we need to eat less, there's more necessity for the foods we consume to be extra nutrient-dense. Even the healthiest of older people have a lower intake of nutrients, and deficiencies are common, especially in current or former smokers. After about age 60 we're less able to absorb and fully use minerals and vitamins.

In studies of older people in care homes, eating a limited range of foods has been connected with under-nutrition, but this is also connected with changes in the gut microbiome (see page 221).

TIP: If you count calories, 1,800 calories a day is suggested as the right amount for moderately active women to age well, and 2,400 for men.

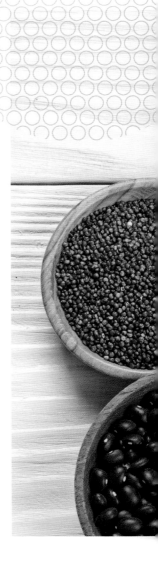

RIGHT: Legumes are nutrient-dense, a useful prebiotic and a good source of the fibre we need to stay healthy into older age.

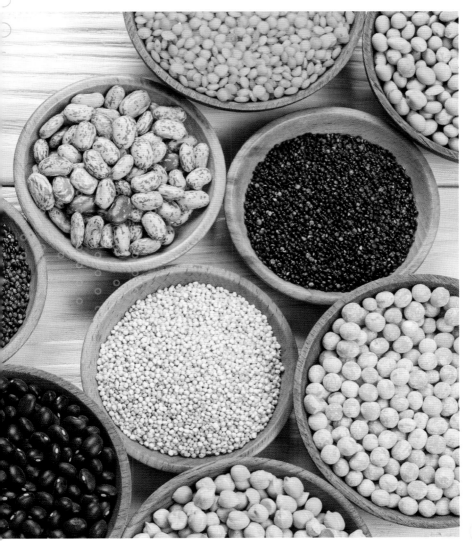

Microbial richness in the gut correlates with healthy and well-functioning body systems. When the diet is limited, the microbiota – the community of bacteria in the gut – collapses. A reduction in the diversity of gut bacteria has been linked with immune problems, inflammatory conditions and obesity, as well as with frailty in older age and triggering disease development. It may contribute to our

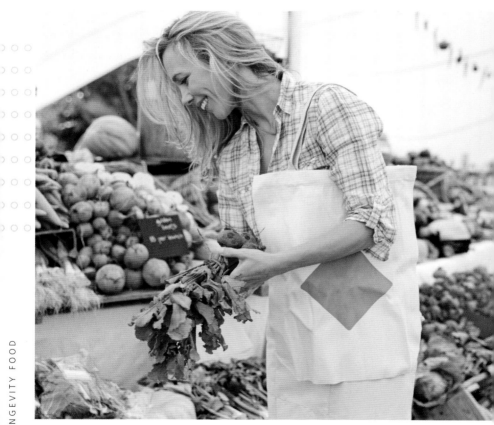

ABOVE: Eating as wide a variety of seasonal vegetables as possible is one of the habits of long-lived people across the globe.

GOOD-FOOD PRINCIPLES

In order to feel energized
and help you to remain
active into older age, eat:

- Foods that are nutrionally
  dense
- Lots of plants
- Plenty of variety
- Slowly
- In company with others

discovered common dietary features in such diverse locations and populations as Okinawa in Japan, Sardinia in Italy and a Seventh Day Adventist community in Loma Linda, California. They all ate a plant-based diet majoring in legumes for main courses. There were other healthy plant-based additions in each location – nuts in California, turmeric in Japan, whole grains and red wine in Sardinia.

Plants are, of course, really old in themselves. Human life developed in areas where plants were able to flourish, and we were eating them long before we discovered fire, hunting, farming and animal husbandry. Our metabolism and physiology are primed to thrive when we eat masses of vegetables because that's the way our species adapted to survive.

The other common denominator of long-lived communities around the globe is the way they eat – stopping what they're doing and gathering as a family or community to spend time around a table, enjoying the company. This is slow eating, which values ingredients, recipes and cooking as something worth talking about, sharing and spending time over. This is food that carries our history, culture and memory and is deeply rooted in a place.

Eating in this way gives us a taste education. We start to trust our taste buds, rather than product packaging or the latest diet guru, to tell us what a healthy meal is. As older people, the

waning ability to absorb protein and even to developing Alzheimer's. Happily, as soon as we start introducing more foods into our diet daily, the gut flora flourish again, and good health resumes. The best way to maintain microbial diversity – and robust health – is to eat as wide a variety of foods as you can most days. Or investigate poo transplants… (Really. Look it up online).

People who live longer tend to share characteristics, wherever in the world they live. When the US National Institute of Aging sponsored research into the regions where people lived longest and with least disease, journalist Dan Buettner

WHO counsels, it's our job to transfer our food culture, health knowledge and cooking skills down the generations, in order to help our children, their children and the wider community to live longer, healthier lives. We are the custodians of health and longevity.

Benefits of good food as we age

Staying healthy into and through older age is as easy as eating well. A diet rich in nutrients from diverse plant foods, whole grains and healthy fats reduces the risk of contracting the most common diseases affecting older people. Heart disease, stroke, diabetes, osteoporosis and cancer are all influenced by diet. Because the chronic degenerative diseases that have a debilitating effect on us in older age begin earlier in life, starting to eat well as young adults ensures we pass through the older decades in better health. And as older people, it's our job to pass on healthy eating habits to our children and grandchildren – food preferences and habits tend to be formed in infancy and are very much influenced by family and culture.

As we age, diet is as important to how we feel emotionally as well as physically – the same foods that protect our heart and circulation, bones and joints, teeth and oral health protect against depression, anxiety (and Alzheimer's). The Mental Health Foundation in the UK found that almost two-thirds of people who eat fresh vegetables, fruit and salad don't report daily mental-health problems; whereas people who do report problems tend to eat less healthily. Omega-3 fatty acids seem to play a particularly effective role in making us feel more mentally stable, as do foods that promote balance in the gut: the fibre in vegetables, fruit and whole grains, and the probiotics in yogurt and

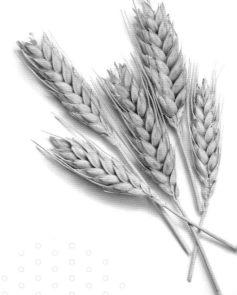

RIGHT: Whole grains are rich in B vitamins and fibre because they contain the entire grain kernel. They also have a fuller flavour and texture.

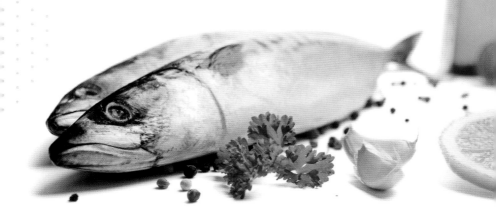

ABOVE: Oily fish support heart health, brain function, good vision and help keep the joints mobile; they are a key source of omega-3 fatty acids.

fermented foods. The gut is in constant communication with the brain via neural pathways activated by good gut bacteria, and it also makes up a huge part of our immune system – there are more immune cells in our intestines than in the rest of the body. The inflammation that plays a role in many of the diseases of ageing, and in depression and hormonal disorders, may also be triggered by malfunctioning microbiota in the gut. Eating well equals a balanced microbiota, equals better immunity and less inflammation – the recipe for healthy ageing.

THE REWARDS FROM EATING GOOD FOOD

As we age, good food:

- Reduces risk of the most common diseases affecting older people, all of which are diet-affected, including heart disease, stroke, diabetes, osteoporosis and cancer.
- Protects bones and joints, teeth and oral health.
- Benefits mood and mental health.
- Maintains a healthy immune system.
- Keeps cases of chronic inflammation in check.

What we need more of with age

There are crucial nutrients associated with a healthy life as we get older. No one food contains them all — there's no single longevity meal or ingredient. By taking a single nutrient out of context we miss out on the synergistic magic that occurs in nature when biologically active chemicals meet and mingle, triggering healing processes not yet understood by science.

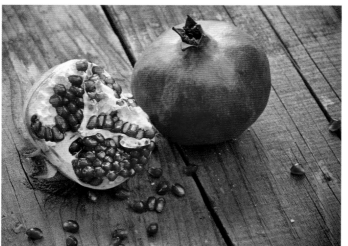

LEFT: Pomegranates contain potent antioxidant polyphenols that seem to protect against many diseases of ageing, including of the heart and blood vessels.

Antioxidants

These help to repair cell damage and can reduce the risk of heart disease, some cancers, Alzheimer's and cataracts. They are especially important for smokers, who have been shown to consume significantly fewer fruit and vegetables than non-smokers. Antioxidants found in plants – vitamins C and E, carotenoids, flavonoids, phenols, tannins, lignans – may help explain the remarkable disease-busting properties of plants. The same active ingredients account for the deliciousness of these foods to palate and eye, contributing the green, yellow, red and purple pigments, and the mouth-watering taste of everything from the tartness of grapefruit to the bite of garlic and the astringency of tea or cranberries. If we eat a good number of different fruits and vegetables, we consume thousands of antioxidants each day.

From: vegetables and fruit, whole grains, nuts and seeds, herbs and spices, black and green tea, coffee, chocolate and cocoa, red wine.

Omega-3 fats

Long-chain essential fatty acids, such as docosahexaenoic acid (DHA) and eicosapentaenoic acid (EPA), keep brain and eyes sharp and protect against heart disease (particularly after a heart attack). They boost general strength and mobility while protecting immunity and warding off depression. Omega-3s may guard against inflammation and help manage rheumatoid arthritis and tender joints and muscles, and they have been associated with reduced risk of developing dementia.

From: oily fish, including salmon, mackerel and sardines; walnuts and flaxseed (these contain alpha-linolenic acid (ALA), which the body has to convert into DHA or EPA, making them less potent).

RIGHT: Whole-wheat grains are complex carbohydrates that break down slowly, releasing sugar into the bloodstream steadily through the day.

Fibre

People who eat the most fibre have a reduced risk of cardiovascular disease. It also keeps the digestive system working smoothly, blood-sugar levels steady and protects against type-2 diabetes, obesity and some cancers. Many older people don't get the recommended daily amount, which is 30g. Prebiotic-rich fibre-filled vegetables, such as leeks, onions and asparagus, help maintain healthy gut flora.

Fibre is often confused with carbohydrates, which have a bad reputation, but complex carbohydrates are rich in fibre and nutrients. The body absorbs them slowly. They keep us feeling satisfied for hours, lift mood and speed recovery after a workout. Complex carbohydrates include unprocessed grains such as oats, quinoa and brown rice, legumes such as lentils and chickpeas, broccoli and sweet potatoes, bananas and berries, and plain yogurt. Aim for these to make up around a third of your diet.

From: vegetables and fruit, legumes, whole grains.

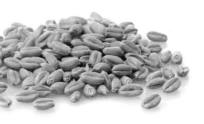

Calcium

We lose bone mass as we age, especially after the menopause, thanks to the reduction in bone-protecting oestrogen. Bearing in mind that we absorb it less well as we get older, including adequate calcium in our diet is vital. As well as protecting bones and teeth, calcium regulates nerve and muscle function and aids blood clotting. It's absorbed most effectively with vitamin D (both calcium and vitamin D are found in milk).

From: dairy produce, fish with edible bones, dark leafy greens, legumes, nuts, fortified foods. (Watch the caffeine, which reduces absorption.)

ß vitamins

B vitamins are responsible for energy production and creating red blood cells, maintaining a healthy nervous system and hormonal balance, and aiding concentration. The combination of B6, B12 and folate (also called folic acid) protects the heart and reduces the risk of stroke, dementia and memory loss, and may help counter depression.

Vitamin B12 absorption is a highly complex process that often becomes less efficient with age. In healthy adults, about half of the B12 in ingested food is absorbed into the body, but loss of function in the stomach, pancreas or

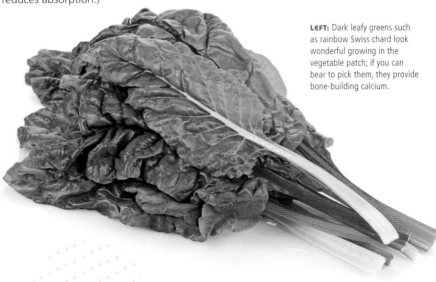

LEFT: Dark leafy greens such as rainbow Swiss chard look wonderful growing in the vegetable patch; if you can bear to pick them, they provide bone-building calcium.

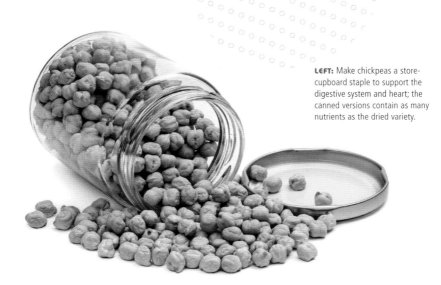

LEFT: Make chickpeas a store-cupboard staple to support the digestive system and heart; the canned versions contain as many nutrients as the dried variety.

small intestine can impair absorption and can lead to a B12 deficiency. Deficiencies in other B vitamins that interact with vitamin B12 may also contribute to age-related cognitive decline. Older people with low levels of B vitamins have noticeably more neurological problems (such as memory issues) and are at risk of anaemia.

From: beans, poultry, fish, fortified foods (B6); fish, poultry, meat, eggs, dairy, fortified foods, yeast extract (B12); spinach, liver, beans, lentils, fortified foods, yeast extract (folate); peas, fruit, eggs, whole grains, liver, fortified foods (B1); milk, eggs, rice, fortified foods (B2).

Vitamin D

This is required for healthy bones and muscles and to help calcium absorption. Deficiency is common in older people, especially women, leading to depleted muscle strength (and possibly depleted neuromuscular function), and is associated with falls and fractures. Meta-analysis studies show a correlation between those with the lowest levels of vitamin D and an increase in mortality from all causes, and cardiovascular death. Up your levels and you're less likely to suffer heart disease, high blood pressure, type-2 diabetes, Alzheimer's, some cancers and osteoporosis.

Already problematic in the winter months, when the sun doesn't contain enough ultraviolet B (UVB) radiation for our skin to manufacture vitamin D, we often don't expose ourselves to enough sunlight for the process to take place (at least 20 minutes a day) at other times of the year, either. In this case, food and supplements become our main sources. This vitamin becomes even more important in older age, especially if we have darker skin. Older skin is less efficient at synthesizing vitamin D, and we're less likely to get the opportunity if we spend more sedentary time indoors or prefer not to expose our skin to the sun.

From: sunlight, eggs, oily fish, fortified foods; a daily supplement of 10mcg is recommended in winter.

Probiotics and prebiotics

The live micro-organisms in probiotics (the very word suggests longevity, deriving from the Latin and Greek "for life") boost the health of the gut and immunity.

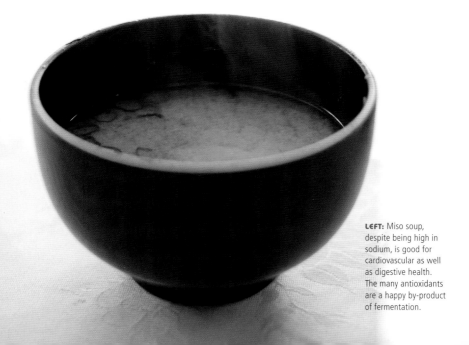

LEFT: Miso soup, despite being high in sodium, is good for cardiovascular as well as digestive health. The many antioxidants are a happy by-product of fermentation.

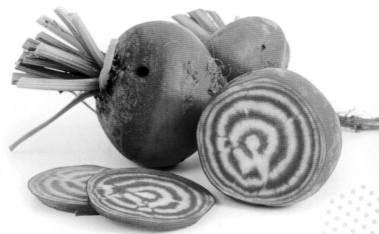

RIGHT: The betalain pigments in the beetroot contribute its antioxidant and anti-inflammatory properties. They also help rid the body of toxins by making them soluble in water.

The body becomes less able to fight disease with age (immunosenescense) and a number of studies in older people show that probiotics boost immunity and may reduce the duration of winter infections. Other studies in older people show they can counter under-nutrition and constipation and promote calcium absorption. Prebiotics stimulate the body's natural probiotic bacteria.

From: yogurt and fermented foods such as sauerkraut, kimchi, kefir, miso (probiotics); onions, garlic, Jerusalem artichokes, chicory (prebiotics).

Magnesium

Essential for healthy bones, cells and nerves, magnesium also protects cardiovascular health and regulates blood sugar. A deficit of this mineral in older people (which can result from under-nutrition and gut problems) has been implicated in the ageing process and with cardiovascular and neuromuscular disorders, hormonal problems and Alzheimer's. Magnesium aids the absorption of calcium and vitamin D.

From: dark leafy greens, nuts and seeds, milk, whole grains, broccoli and spinach, beetroot, legumes.

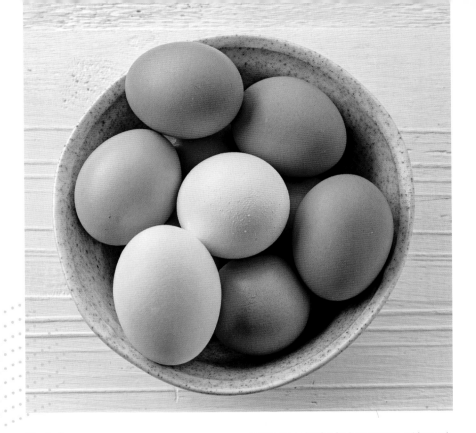

Protein

We lose muscle mass as we age (a process known as sarcopenia) because the body becomes less good at turning protein into muscle. As a result, wounds don't heal as quickly, skin is less elastic and it's harder to fight infection and recover from illness. Older people need more protein than younger adults, but data shows the average daily protein

ABOVE: The perfect fast food: easy to store, quick to cook, packed with nutrients – and delicious.

intake of many older people is well above the recommended requirement. Animal protein also delivers folic acid and B12.

From: eggs, lean meat, fish, dairy, nuts, legumes.

> *"One cannot think well, love well, sleep well, if one has not dined well."*
>
> **VIRGINIA WOOLF**

PLEASURE

Most of all we need more pleasure as we head into our later decades and recognize we have fewer years in which to experience all the good things the world has to offer. There's an amazing amount of pleasure to be had in food, and not just the sensory pleasure of the taste, smell and mouth feel, or the practical pleasure of cooking, or the social pleasure of sharing. A huge amount of pleasure comes from knowing the provenance of food – the tomato that fell from the vine outside the back door from being so ripe, the lamb

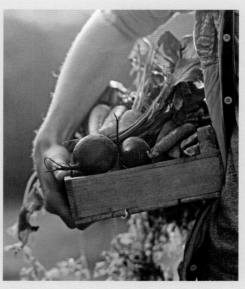

fed on rain-soaked grass that would be a bramble patch without its presence, the loaf from the baker who got up at 2am to start his day. It's the pleasure of being part of the circle of life, what the writer and environmentalist Wendell Berry refers to as eating with the "fullest pleasure" because it expresses our connection with the world and the mystery of our dependence on "creatures we did not make and powers we cannot comprehend". That awareness is common to the food cultures of the most long-lived communities around the globe.

ABOVE: The pleasure of growing your own food only increases with age, as we learn what thrives in our particular climate and soil.

Longer-life foods

The key to good eating as we age is diversity – of colours on the plate, types of foods and nutrients. If we eat the same foods day-in day-out, it can lead to decreased nutritional status and a depleted gut biome, which triggers many of the ailments associated with ageing.

Here are some of the key life-enhancing foods we need more of on most days. Many of them are plants. Plant foods contain such good nutritional properties that long-term vegetarians (think over 17 years) have a life expectancy almost four years longer than meat eaters. We can benefit from all that botanical diversity by eating more plants.

TIP: Eating ten portions of fruit and vegetables a day could cut your risk of dying prematurely by 31 per cent, found researchers from Imperial College London.

Chickpeas

Part of the human diet for nine thousand years, chickpeas are packed with antioxidants, fantastic for protein and folate, and have enough fibre to help prevent constipation, lower cholesterol and keep blood-sugar and insulin levels stable. They contain good amounts of calcium and magnesium for bones, too. In Ayurvedic medicine, chickpeas are valued in older age for supporting the metabolism and building the body, especially in the weak, and are recommended for digestive health.

Oily fish

Of your two to three portions of fish a week, at least one should be oily (salmon, sardines, mackerel, anchovies) to deliver useful calcium if you consume the bones, omega-3 fatty acids and vitamin D. Studies of older people suggest that those who eat plenty of fish show enhanced activity in the memory and emotional areas of the brain and less cognitive decline. Don't eat more than four portions per week because of potential contaminants, such as PCBs (neurological toxins associated with cancer) and

DAILY LONGEVITY FORMULA

- Eat at least five portions of vegetables and fruit, but ten portions if you can (a portion is as much as you can fit in your hand. Fruit juice counts as one portion).

- Use extra-virgin olive oil to aid nutrient absorption (use for dressings, dipping or cooking slowly in the oven, but not for frying or roasting – see page 201). The US Food and Drug Administration (FDA) recommends eating about two tablespoons of olive oil a day for heart health.

- Eat five to six small non-fatty meals – people who do this eat a greater variety of foods and maintain a healthy stable weight.

- Aim for half your plate to be vegetables, fruit, herbs and spices, a quarter whole grains and the final quarter protein, including dairy.

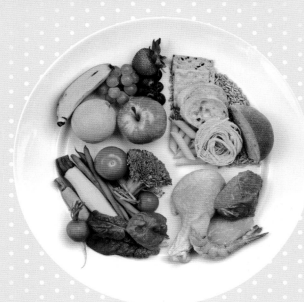

mercury. Small fish lower down the food chain contain fewer contaminants than farmed salmon or larger carnivorous fish, such as tuna.

Garlic

Valued for relaxing and enlarging the blood vessels, improving blood flow and as an anticoagulant, garlic is an aid to cardiovascular health. Two to three cloves daily are associated with reducing risk of heart attack and stroke by a quarter. Garlic has been used since ancient Greek times for its wound-healing properties and ability to bolster the body against stress and increase immunity. It is antimicrobial, antiseptic, antiviral, antifungal and anti-inflammatory and may reduce the frequency and severity of colds. The main active ingredients, including the antiviral agent ajoene, are responsible for the pungent odour and much of the medicinal action.

Nutritionally, garlic delivers calcium and vitamin B6 while boosting vitamin absorption. As a prebiotic, garlic benefits digestion, encouraging the growth of good bacteria in the gut and easing bloating and gas. In culinary amounts, there should be no interaction with blood-thinning or anti-clotting medication, but avoid supplements.

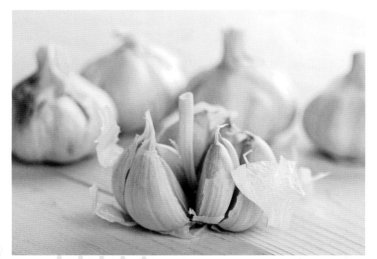

RIGHT: Blueberries have antioxidant and anti-inflammatory properties, and protect the cardiovascular system and cognitive function.

LEFT: A couple of garlic cloves a day benefit the cardiovascular and digestive systems, immunity and detoxification and fight inflammation.

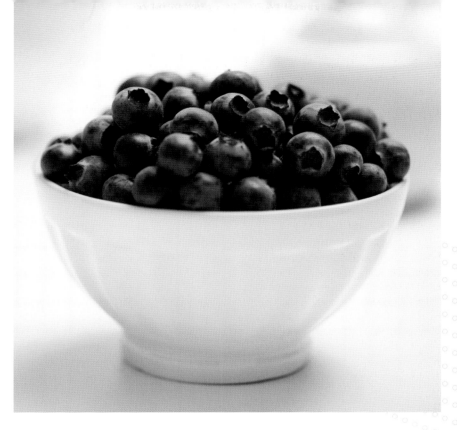

Blueberries

Blueberries have the highest antioxidant count of any fresh fruit, thanks to the constituent phenolic compounds, anthocyanins, which give anti-inflammatory, anti-blood clotting and antibacterial properties. Consumption of half a cup daily (about 30 berries) is said to aid the formation of connective tissue, and strengthen and relax blood vessels, normalizing blood pressure. Other constituents – ellagic acid and pectin – benefit the gastrointestinal system, while tannins act on the urinary tract in a way similar to cranberries to prevent infection. They contain a good amount of fibre, too. Studies on older people have linked consumption of blueberries with short-term memory enhancement.

Apples

Apples contain some of the highest levels of the antioxidant phenolic compound quercetin, which has an anti-inflammatory action, prevents blood from clumping and regulates blood pressure; another flavonoid in apples, phloridzin, supports the lungs. Easy on digestion, apples contain malic and tartaric acids, which reduce acidity and inhibit fermentation in the intestines. The soluble fibre pectin encourages beneficial gut flora to flourish while balancing blood-sugar levels.

Nutritionally, apples provide folate and lots of fibre – just one apple can provide 15 per cent of daily requirements. Research has found cloudy apple juice more beneficial for the heart and lungs than regular apple juice. Apple cider vinegar, considered the essence of youth in some cultures, is thought to ease indigestion and aid calcium absorption.

Ginger

Renowned as a panacea in many Asian traditional healthcare systems, ginger gains its remarkable healing powers (and zingy taste) from the phenolic compound gingerol, which also has pain-killing and antibacterial properties. Ginger root is remarkably rich in antioxidants (only pomegranates and some berries have more). It has an anti-inflammatory action and decreases pain, and may be recommended to relieve the symptoms of arthritis.

Ginger stimulates circulation (try drinking ginger tea if you have poor peripheral circulation and suffer with leg cramps or cold hands and feet) and seems to protect against cardiovascular disease. It may be beneficial in treating dementia, appears to reduce cholesterol and may help to manage diabetes. But it's probably best known for its effect on the gastrointestinal system, encouraging appetite and good digestion, and countering nausea and constipation. It's also a carminative (it helps in releasing wind). Nutritionally, ginger root is a good source of vitamin B6.

Olive oil

The bright star of the Mediterranean diet, olive oil is amazingly good for cardiovascular health – according to one study, increasing your intake of extra-virgin olive oil by 10g a day could reduce your risk of cardiovascular disease by up to 10 per cent. The phenolic compounds in the oil (extra-virgin has most) produce the famed anti-inflammatory, antioxidant and anticoagulant properties, and help blood vessels to relax and dilate, while its oleic acid helps maintain healthy cholesterol levels. The phenolic compounds also seem to benefit bone health. The stinging sensation at the back of the throat in peppery extra-virgin olive oil indicates the presence of oleocanthal, which has pain-relieving and anti-inflammatory powers

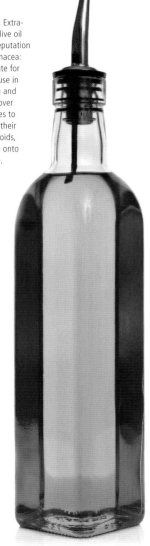

RIGHT: Extra-virgin olive oil has a reputation as a panacea: substitute for butter, use in cooking and drizzle over tomatoes to release their carotenoids, and rub onto dry skin.

WHEN TO REACH FOR OLIVE OIL

To get the most benefit from the health-boosting properties (and delicious taste) of olive oil, choose extra-virgin for making salad dressings and mayonnaise or aioli and for dipping bread; it's also good for slow cooking robust dishes in the oven. Some people prefer not to use olive oil for frying or roasting because it has a low "smoke" point (extra-virgin has the highest of all the olive oils). The polyunsaturated fats that make up around 11 per cent of the total fats in olive oil aren't stable at high temperatures. They can oxidize and form harmful compounds linked with cancer (which is why it's not a good idea to heat wholly polyunsaturated fats, such as sunflower oil). You might like to substitute rapeseed oil, which contains the healthy omega 3, 6 and 9 essential fatty acids of olive oil, but has a high "flash point" that is safe at high temperatures.

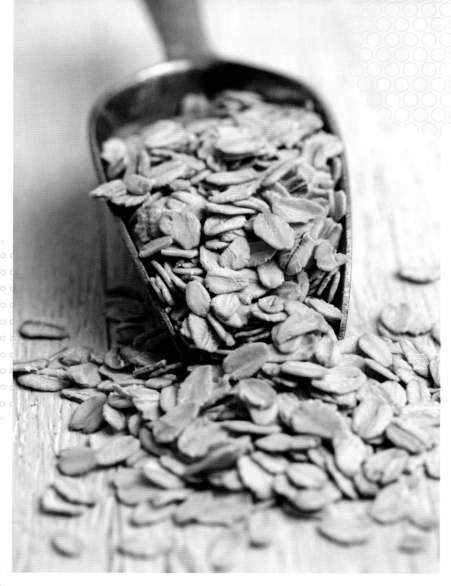

similar to ibuprofen. The constituent unsaturated fatty acid squaline, which occurs in human skin, is thought useful for boosting suppleness and countering environmental damage in older skin. The soothing demulcent properties also suit olive oil to protecting the digestive system (its antimicrobial action can ease gastrointestinal problems), and these softening qualities contribute to its value as a gentle laxative.

Oats

Rich in easily assimilated protein, oats are also a fantastically concentrated source of soluble fibre known as beta-glucan, which lowers cholesterol and can significantly reduce the risk of cardiovascular disease and stroke. This seems especially beneficial for postmenopausal women. The fibre guards against constipation, too, enhances immunity and stabilizes blood-sugar. Antioxidant avenanthramides benefit cardiovascular health, while oats also deliver essential fatty acids, B vitamins, calcium and magnesium. These whole grains are supportive for the nervous system, recommended to ease exhaustion and treat insomnia. Extract of oats has been shown to be useful in helping people quit smoking.

LEFT: Oats regularly appear on lists of must-eat foods for their big hit of vitamins, minerals and antioxidants, soluble fibre and protein.

Eggs

The regenerative food *par excellence*, eggs contain everything necessary to nurture new life. The UN has declared eggs a better source of protein than milk, fish, beef and legumes. Eggs are rich in B vitamins and the yolk includes the choline we need to absorb folate. They contain antioxidants (lutein and zeaxanthin) that alongside omega-3 fatty acids can safeguard eye health and help prevent age-related macular degeneration (AMD), which causes loss of central vision.

As well as memory-protecting choline, eggs contain vitamin D for immunity and calcium absorption, plus the amino acid leucine, necessary for continuing muscle strength and function. Eggs from hens raised on pasture can contain almost ten times as many omega-3 fatty acids (and up to six times more vitamin E) than those from indoor hens.

Walnuts

Prized in Traditional Chinese Medicine as the longevity fruit, walnuts are one of the best sources of antioxidants and are rich in the omega-3 essential fatty acids we need for a healthy brain and heart. Studies suggest that, in improving heart health, they may be as helpful as olive oil – the constituent amino acid L-arginine protects the elasticity of blood vessels, helping to lower blood pressure. Walnuts have been associated with managing levels of cholesterol and supporting a healthy digestive and immune system. They also seem to boost melatonin. Apply walnut oil topically to regenerate dry skin.

Fermented foods

Live yogurt is recommended for the health of the gut and for boosting immunity. While lactose intolerance seems to worsen with age, yogurt remains well tolerated, making it a good way to obtain calcium – there's more calcium in yogurt than in milk. The combination of calcium plus vitamins D and K in milk products supports bone health, while yogurt's B vitamins and omega-3 fatty acids are as welcome as the high amounts of protein. As with eggs, choose produce from animals reared on grass for the richest supply of vitamins and healthy fats.

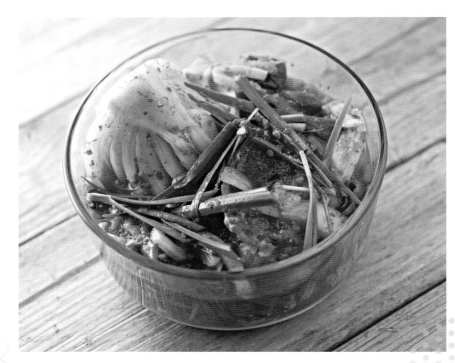

Other traditional fermented foods – sauerkraut, kimchi, kefir, miso – can be incredibly helpful for digestive health. When vegetables or fruit ferment, naturally occurring micro-organisms convert their sugar and starch into lactic acid. This preserves the food and gives the telltale tartness (it's the same *Lactobacillus* bacteria found in yogurt). The fermentation process increases the availability of vitamins and minerals and because the food has already started breaking down, they are easier for the gut to extract. The pH of these foods helps make the digestive tract more acidic, which benefits the gastric juices, which trigger the release of enzymes in the pancreas, gallbladder and stomach that we need to digest food. This is especially helpful if our natural production of digestive enzymes has declined with age. So the message is more nutrients, easier digestion, healthier gut.

LEFT: A side helping of fermented foods adds tang and taste to a meal, while the beneficial bacteria from the fermentation process boost digestion and immunity.

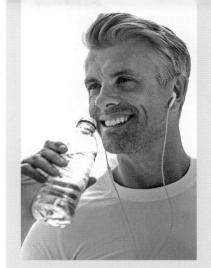

WATER

Our thirst sensation declines as we age even if we stay healthy, making dehydration a distinct possibility. Water is essential to the health of all the body's systems. It optimizes digestion, ensures our metabolism and mood stay stable, and hydrates the brain for better mental performance. Aim to drink six to eight glasses daily – at least 1.5 litres (2½ pints) – spread out through the day, more if it's warm and humid or while exercising.

Magic beans

The broad, or fava, bean is one of the oldest plants used for food. It has been eaten for some ten thousand years – before there were grains there were beans. Since prehistoric times and across civilizations it has been associated with rebirth and magical growth, immortality and the potential for communion with other worlds. It's one of the best foods as we age, containing B vitamins, folate, fibre and protein, and is being investigated as a way of encouraging the manufacture of dopamine in Parkinson's patients.

The bean is perhaps associated with prolonged life because it arrives early in the growing season and, once dried, lasts seemingly forever, maintaining the potential to spring to life after a good soaking and boiling. Legend tells of beans sprouting after three or four thousand years. In ancient Egypt, the hollow pods were considered a passageway to the other world and were buried alongside the deceased, while in ancient Greece Pythagoras thought beans contained the essence of man; a bean was a container for the soul after death awaiting potential regeneration.

The bean is a potent symbol of life to come – plant just one and the return may be a thousand-fold. No wonder it's this bean that Jack casts out of the window, waking next morning to find a giant beanstalk that leads him to the upper world and the treasure of the golden goose. Full of riches for the gardener, too, the bean replenishes the soil as it grows, taking nitrogen from the air and fixing it into the earth, preparing a bed so that plants that take root there next year will also thrive. An old bean is in charge of future fortune, worn as a lucky charm and baked into the divination cake of Twelfth Night – whoever receives the slice with the hidden bean will be King of the Revels. Umberto Eco tells of the bean bringing fortune and longevity to an

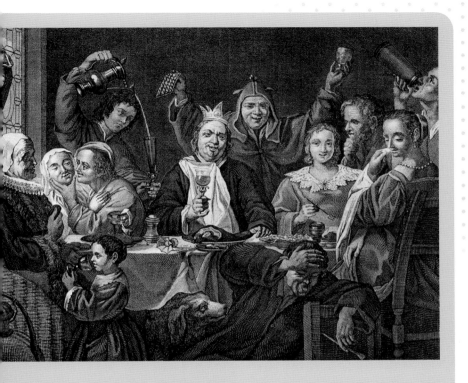

entire continent. From the time beans arrived in Europe, cultivated since the 10th century, they provided a stable source of protein that ensured the population became healthier and lived longer – long enough to populate the continent and ensure a renaissance of church, commerce and industry that in turn sent out ships to conquer a new continent on the other side of the Atlantic.

ABOVE: Twelfth-Night revels in 1640 feature games and guising; fortunes can be made or reversed according to the vagaries of chance and a lucky bean.

Bulgarian longevity recipe

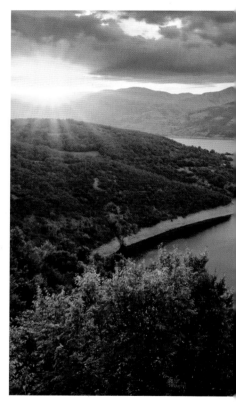

In the early 20th century, Russian Nobel-prize-winning scientist Ilya Metchnikov at the Pasteur Institute looked at which country produced most centenarians. Out of the 38 countries studied, Bulgaria stood out, with four people in every 1,000 aged 100 or over. He ascribed the high number of centenarians to consumption of yogurt, a Bulgarian invention legendarily attributed to the Thracian people (in Roman times) carrying sheep's milk around in lambskin bags warmed by the body. The bacteria that gives the unique taste is *Lactobacillus bulgaricus*, a naturally occurring strain that only thrives in Bulgaria. It is found in the soil, tree blossom, bark and even ant hills in ecologically pristine regions such as the Rhodope Mountains in the south of the country, said to be home to the world's highest concentration of centenarians. This may have as much to do with the pristine environment of the remote region and a diet rich in fresh organic vegetables and herbs as with the yogurt (consumption halved with the decline of the Russian empire).

Longevity here may also have something to do with the value put on community, the active manual labour and hill walking, and a stress-free lifestyle that values sleep and rest. Then the genes of long-lived ancestors are preserved in

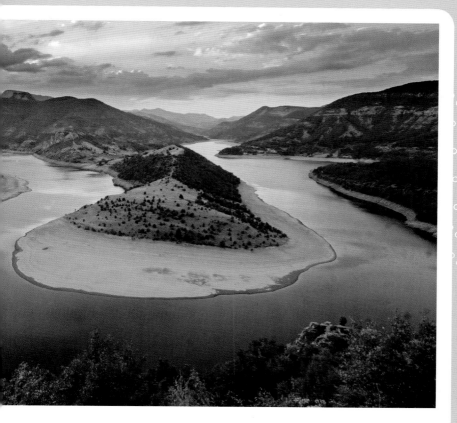

a remote region. Researchers who've been following the very old people in the area for decades point at similar pockets of extreme age in other isolated communities in the Caucasus Mountains, Himalayas and Andes.

ABOVE: The Rhodope Mountains in southern Bulgaria – the reputed birthplace of Orpheus, and a place so remote that his descendants are said to live there still.

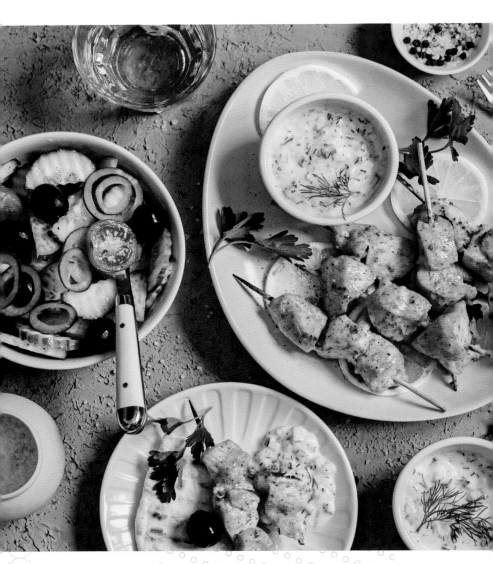

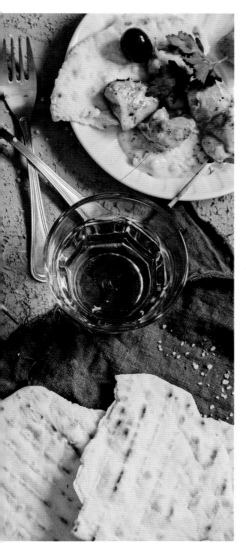

What's the best diet?

Alkaline, 5:2, low-carb, low-fat, high-protein, raw – it's all so confusing. It's easy to shift from diet to diet, from latest wonder gadget to wellness guru, and fail to keep it up long enough to see the fabled results. But at the (healthy) heart of most diets that work is the same formula – eat more plant-based foods and a greater variety of foods, and consume fewer manufactured foods. This has been shown to boost longevity and lower risk of cardiovascular disease, diabetes, cancer and Alzheimer's. It's one of the best diets for heart health and for countering inflammation.

This diet is similar to the traditional Mediterranean diet, which is high in nutrients from plenty of fresh plant foods and whole grains, legumes and nuts, fish, small amounts of lean meat and a little dairy, with olive as the main oil and moderate consumption of wine. People who eat this way tend to live longer – whether they're in the Med or not.

This way of eating shares traits with the traditional Japanese diet, which is high in nutrients from eating plenty of fresh plant foods and whole grains, legumes, fish, small amounts of meat – but this time hardly any dairy and lots of soy, fermented

LEFT: The Mediterranean diet: plenty of vegetables and fruit, fish and legumes, but above all plenty of taste.

foods such as miso, and sea vegetables. People who eat this way live longer *en masse* than anywhere else in the world, though the beneficial effects have not been replicated outside Japan.

What can we draw from this? Both are traditional diets with no manufactured foods. When Mediterranean and Japanese people eat fast food, their health and longevity decline. So the point is to eat close to the bottom of the food chain and choose foods our great-great-grandparents knew. The most important part of a healthy diet is being able to stick to it forever, which is maybe why traditional ways of eating pass healthy habits down the generations.

The ultimate "only eat what your ancestors would recognize as food" diet is the paleo diet – the diet of those ancestors living 40 generations ago. This means consuming mostly vegetables, lean meat, fish, eggs, nuts, fruit and plant oils – no grains or legumes, no dairy or other cultivated foods. Paleo meat is raised in the traditional way, on pasture and forage crops (rather than being fed soya-based feeds and cereals), making it lower in saturated fat and higher in omega-3 fatty acids and conjugated linoleic acid (CLA, found in dairy produce and animal fats), B vitamins, calcium and magnesium. The verdict seems to be that since so few people eat this way – it's not a traditional diet sustained over recent generations – there's no good evidence to support its use generally, let alone in older age, and many dietitians consider it foolish to cut out such high-nutrient foods as legumes, grains and dairy.

EAT SUSTAINABLY

Processed food and meal-delivery apps are wiping out local food cultures – and since this way of eating tends to contain more sugar, salt and unhealthy fat than home-cooked food, it's harming our health, too. Refined foods are destroying environments around the world as traditional ways of farming are ditched to cultivate crops such as palm oil and crop-based animal feeds.

The sustainable food movement champions food that's created, sold and eaten in ways that benefit society, husbandry and health. As older people we tend to be closer to the food traditions that sustained our ancestors in the places we call home. We can do our bit by being standard bearers for local, seasonal produce, by passing on food customs and by sharing ways of cooking time-honoured dishes from scratch.

WHAT TO EAT?

For a more youthful heart, veins, joints, bones, muscles, brain, hormones, prostate, skin and hair, mood and sleep, it's probably best to eat:

• Lots of vegetables and fruit (make them deep green and brightly coloured, and include some cooked tomatoes), garlic, whole grains, legumes, herbs and spices, olive oil.

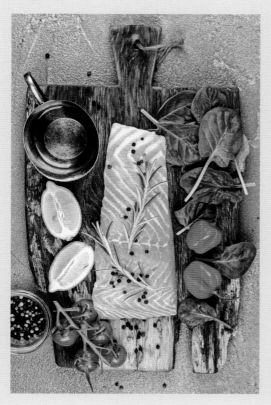

• Moderate amounts of oily fish, nuts and seeds, live yogurt and fermented foods, eggs, lean meat, dark chocolate.

• Drink water, green and black tea, coffee, milk and a glass of red wine with meals.

LEFT: Health on a platter: oily fish, herbs and spices, olive oil, fruit and plenty of vegetables.

What we need less of with age

The WHO states that our first line of attack in preventing heart disease and stroke should be to modify our diet, using food – not drugs – to keep cholesterol and blood pressure at healthy levels.

That means looking at how much salt, sugar and saturated fat we eat. Even modest reductions can have a substantial effect. But let's not get too obsessed with cutting stuff out. In communities where people tend to live longer lives, eating is not about avoidance, it's about addition – more nutrient-dense foods, more time to savour them and more people to enjoy them with.

Salt
Eat less salt and you reduce your risk of heart disease and stroke. Simple. Aim for less than one teaspoon per day – not so simple when 75 per cent of salt in our diet is found in manufactured foods.

Saturated fat and trans-fats
When we eat saturated fat, the liver turns it into blood cholesterol, which causes the blood vessels to narrow or become blocked, making heart disease and stroke more likely. Saturated fat also contributes to inflammation. In the West, many older adults eat more than the recommended amount of saturated fats, which is 20g per day for women,

30g for men. Full-fat dairy produce, meat and coconut oil contain saturated fat, but we're more likely to eat it in processed foods, which include most supermarket pastries, pies, biscuits, cakes, confectionery, snack foods, ready meals and fried foods. These are also our most likely sources of trans-fats (look for "hydrogenated fats" on labels). These hard fats are a by-product of processing and frying and raise cholesterol levels and triglycerides, increasing the risk of coronary heart disease more than saturated fats. Don't reach instead for foods marked "low-fat" because they're likely to contain sugar. Margarine is tricky; avoid the old-fashioned solid ones, which may contain trans-fats, and choose softer spreads based on healthier unsaturated fats. Often, a drizzle of olive oil will taste better.

Sugar
The WHO recommends that sugar should form less than 5 per cent of our daily food intake (definitely no more than 10 per cent). That's because it can lead to increased risk of heart disease, diabetes

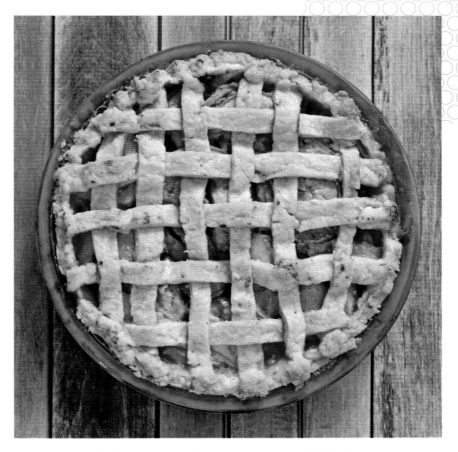

ABOVE: Make it yourself when you crave a treat; it's so satisfying to serve a home-baked pie still warm from the oven.

TIP: All the bad stuff is in manufactured foods, from biscuits to pies to snacks to ready meals. Cook from scratch and you're less likely to meet them.

and obesity. It also increases inflammation. Ingredients ending in "ose" (maltose, dextrose, glucose, fructose, sucrose) are secret sugars. Sugar-free products may be even worse – artificial sweeteners such as aspartame (E951), saccharin (E954) and acesulfame K (E950) have been linked with health concerns.

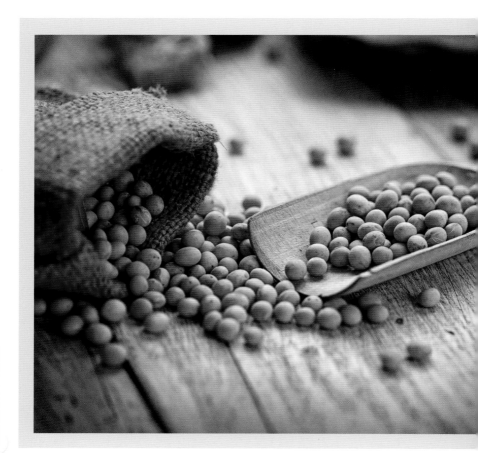

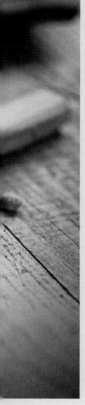

SOY

Soy products contain isoflavones, plant chemicals with a structure similar to oestrogen, and although they're often recommended to help relieve menopausal symptoms, the results of studies are not consistent. After looking at the evidence, the American Association of Clinical Endocrinologists (AACE) states that their effect on relieving menopausal symptoms is inconsistent and has not been shown to lessen hot flushes. The results on menopausal bone loss were mixed.

There's controversy about whether the kind of soy found in soya milk, tofu and other unfermented products is actually beneficial. In places where it's part of the traditional diet, soy is eaten fermented (such as in tempeh or miso). Unfermented, it has been linked with the growth of breast-cancer cells, and the AACE advises against using soy-based treatments if you (or your family) have a history of heart disease or blood clots or hormone-sensitive cancers (such as breast or ovarian).

Soy protein used to be thought useful for lowering cholesterol, blood pressure and other risk factors for heart disease and stroke. But the American Heart Association says soy protein has no observable benefit on cardiovascular health. That said, tofu and other soy products may be beneficial if they replace burgers and such like, which contain lots of saturated fat.

LEFT: Soy beans have the most nutritional benefit when consumed as whole foods and fermented rather than processed.

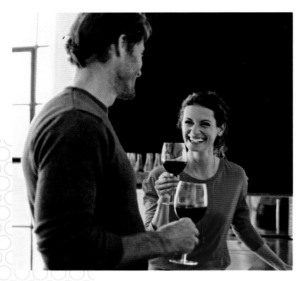

LEFT: Red wine has been linked with more health benefits than other forms of alcohol, perhaps because of the plant compounds it contains, such as antioxidant resveratrol.

RIGHT: The third day of creation, when the earth brings forth grass, "herb-yielding seed" and fruit trees.

Processed meat

That means cured meats, including bacon and ham, sausage and hot dogs. The WHO says processed meat ranks alongside smoking as a cause of cancer, thanks to the nitrite/nitrates used in the preserving process. Aim for less than 70g per day – 1½ sausages or 3 slices of ham.

Red meat

Most research on health and meat finds that the more red meat we eat, the more prone we are to die sooner than those who rarely eat it – 26 per cent more likely, according to one study of half a million people. Risks are increased for all causes of death by disease, including heart disease and stroke, cancer and diseases of the kidneys, liver and respiratory system. As with processed meat, aim for less than 70g per day.

Alcohol

One small glass of red wine a day is good. Its antioxidant phenols thin the blood, keep the artery walls healthy and lower blood pressure, reducing risk of coronary heart disease, stroke and dementia, while boosting immunity. The health benefits are cancelled if you drink more. The recommended maximum is 14 units a week for men and women, with at least two alcohol-free days a week to allow your system time to recover.

FOOD, CLEAN OR DIRTY?

There's an increasing tendency to talk of food as clean or dirty, moralizing about the contents of our plates. As we get older, the anti-pleasure ethic of the wellness industry, with its focus on the perfect and perfectable body, can seem quite unhelpful, even downright depressing. Early religious texts set up the notion that eating plants is clean (and therefore everything else dirty). In *Genesis* (1:29) God says: "Behold, I have given you every herb bearing seed, which is upon the face of all the earth, and every tree, in which is the fruit of a tree yielding seed; to you it shall be for meat." Later he gives us birds and fish. Only after the flood are we allowed meat. From Hinduism, Buddhism and Jainism comes the notion of karma and reincarnation – if we live a pure life, following the principles of vegetarianism and food-prep rules, including breaking earthenware vessels after use, we ascend to a greater life after death. If you don't live your regular life by religious principles, you might not want to live your food life this way, where plant equals purity and animal, sin. Adam lived to 930 despite disobeying God's law.

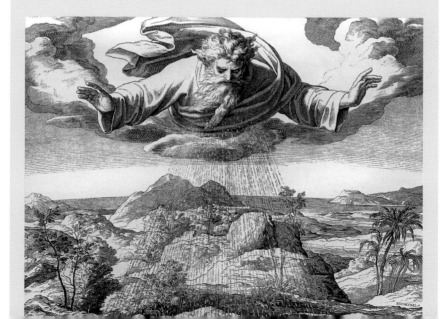

Healthy digestion

The digestive system can get sluggish as we age, leading to problems including bloating and constipation. Without a well-functioning gut, we don't extract maximum nutrients from foods.

THE DIGESTIVE SYSTEM

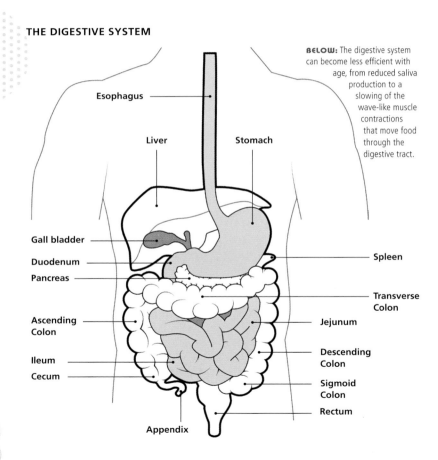

BELOW: The digestive system can become less efficient with age, from reduced saliva production to a slowing of the wave-like muscle contractions that move food through the digestive tract.

Esophagus

Liver

Stomach

Gall bladder

Duodenum

Pancreas

Ascending Colon

Ileum

Cecum

Appendix

Spleen

Transverse Colon

Jejunum

Descending Colon

Sigmoid Colon

Rectum

Since a large proportion of the immune system is found in the lining of the gastrointestinal tract and serotonin is manufactured in the gut, the health of this body system is key to keeping every part of us healthy and feeling well balanced.

The gut is a world all on its own, a microbiome, with its own population – up to a thousand species of bacteria. They develop in us from birth and support healthy digestion and elimination, including the take-up of nutrients from food, while safeguarding immunity. The richer and more stable this micro-world inside us, the more likely we are to stay healthy and live long. The usual advice is to eat a good diet with plenty of fibre and variety, take lots of exercise and get proper relaxation.

The microbiome doesn't like stress or high blood pressure and is upset by antibiotics and manufactured foods. An overload of sugar disrupts the microbial balance (bloating or constipation is a sign). The ageing process seems to deplete the complex blend of bacteria in the microbiome – it's affected negatively by a slowing down in lifestyle and increased illness and medication – and

when that happens, immune-related and inflammatory diseases and obesity become more likely.

There are easy ways to safeguard the health of the microbiome and digestive system. First, eat more unprocessed plants and foods that contain gut-friendly ingredients – oats for a gentle form of fibre, leeks and onions for the inulin that feeds good gut bacteria, herbs and spices including ginger, turmeric and cumin, mint and fennel that soothe and have a carminative (wind-relieving) action. Drink more water to keep digestion moving. Traditionally fermented foods, such as sauerkraut or kimchi, are rich in probiotic bacteria that help to maintain or restore healthy intestinal flora (see page 205).

We nurture the whole digestive process by paying it more attention. Digestion begins with the senses, which react to the smell and sight of food, triggering the flow of the saliva we need to start breaking it down (we lose saliva as we age). Slow and mindful eating allows time for the senses to get to work, and also encourages us to chew more slowly to break down foods before they travel further into the digestive system.

TIP: Keep a food diary to link how and what you eat to digestive symptoms. It can help you highlight trigger foods and deduce whether taking smaller meals more often benefits digestion.

Physical activity is key – a sedentary life means sedentary digestion – as is reducing unnecessary stress. Exercise benefits digestion because when we're fit, the body doesn't need to borrow blood from the digestive system in order to do its work. If we're less fit, the body slows digestion to feed the muscles and lungs. That's why we should wait a couple of hours after eating before exercising. Studies suggest that exercise also alters the bacterial composition of the gut, and that athletes have both a more diverse range of bacteria in the gut and more in total. Yoga has always been valued for safeguarding digestion, both by stimulating the organs of the digestive system to ensure adequate breakdown of food and transportation of waste through the upper and lower intestines, and by switching on the "rest and digest" nervous system.

TIP: Stop eating before you feel full. Studies of long-lived communities identified eating until 80 per cent full as a trait. Body-awareness activities, such as yoga, qigong and the Feldenkrais Method, tune us in to the body's interior signals.

INFLAMMATION

When the body is damaged, the immune system triggers an inflammatory response, which helps combat infection and kick-start tissue repair. As we age we're more prone to living with chronic inflammation that extends beyond a particular area of damage. It seems to contribute to (and be a symptom of) most diseases of older age, including heart disease, type-2 diabetes, cancer, Alzheimer's and autoimmune conditions. In a study of three thousand civil servants in the UK, having elevated markers of inflammation seemed to increase the likelihood of cardiovascular disease and death. Conversely, lower levels correlated with healthy ageing. Inflammation is made worse if we're sedentary (and if we train intensively) and by stress, smoking and drinking too much. It's been linked to a reduction in levels and numbers of bacteria in our gut microbiome, which gives a clue to ways to guard against and treat inflammation – a healthy diet is an anti-inflammatory diet. That means eating plenty of antioxidant-loaded and healthy-fat-loaded vegetables and fruit, herbs and spices, whole grains, legumes, nuts and seeds and oily fish.

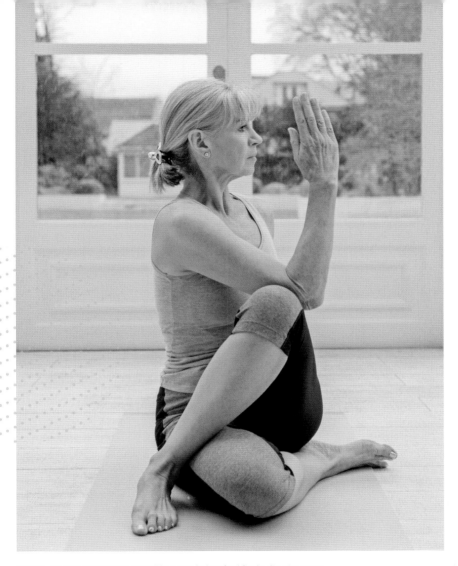

ABOVE: Yoga twisting postures are well known to be beneficial for the digestive system.

Easy twist

Yoga twists work by squeezing and releasing the organs and muscles around the abdomen. This kneading action allows a fresh flow of oxygenated blood into the tissues every time the squeeze is released and stimulates the digestive tract.

1. Lie on your back, with arms outstretched in line with your shoulders, palms facing down, knees bent and feet in the air. Try to keep your legs together.

2. Breathing out, start taking your knees down toward your right side. Keep both shoulders and arms pinned to the floor. Your legs don't have to touch the floor.

3. As you inhale, engage your abdominal muscles to bring your knees back to centre.

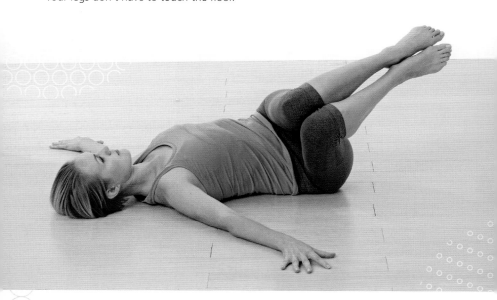

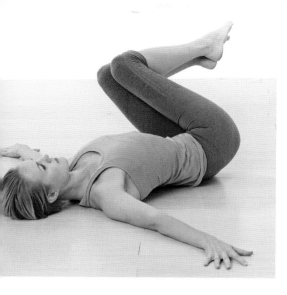

4. As you exhale, drop your knees to the other side, then return to centre on an in-breath. Continue dropping your knees from one side to the other, synchronizing the movements with your breath.

5. Once you've warmed up you might like to drop your knees to the floor and rest in that position, aiming to keep both shoulders down. Look toward your opposite hand, if comfortable. Hold for 30–60 seconds, then activate your abdominal muscles to lift your legs back to centre and repeat to the other side.

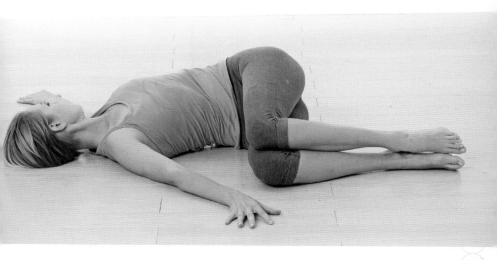

Wind-relieving pose

This aptly named pose, recommended as an Ayurvedic digestive tonic, is useful to relieve constipation, gas and other digestive discomfort.

1. Lie on your back and hug both knees toward your chest. You might like to rock from side to side until you feel more comfortable. Stretch the back of your neck along the floor to release tension in the shoulders (or cushion your head with a folded blanket or towel) and relax your shoulders to the floor. Relax your feet. Hold for up to two minutes, pressing your knees toward your chest as you exhale and releasing with the inhalation. If this is an easy pose, focus on pressing your sitting bones toward the ground.

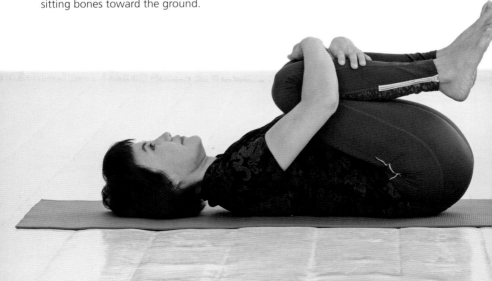

HERBS FOR DIGESTIVE SYMPTOMS

Herbs with a carminative action contain volatile oils that encourage peristalsis, and are useful for relieving wind, bloating and colicky cramping. Take them as teas or use in culinary amounts in cooking:

- **Peppermint:** relaxes the smooth muscles around the intestine, reducing spasms.

- **Fennel:** eases gas, heartburn and bloating, and encourages an appetite.

- **Aniseed:** for painful trapped wind.

- **Lemon balm:** relaxing effect on muscle spasms, and antibacterial too.

- **Chamomile:** useful for colicky spasms and diarrhoea, choose the variety *Matricaria recutita*, or German chamomile.

Fasting

Farmers have always known that periods of malnutrition and starvation don't harm their livestock – in fact, reducing the amount animals are fed (by 30–40 per cent) seems to extend their life (by a third or more).

In people? Well, paleo-eaters would argue that the ancient lifestyle of hunters meant intermittent feast or famine (not three regular meals a day), which led to evolutionary advantages, such as quick-thinking and the ability to move fast and stay alive for longer. The fact remains that restricting calories is the only intervention known to extend life across species.

There's increasing evidence that fasting could be effective in maintaining longevity. While a complete water-only fast should be supervised, and is incredibly difficult to keep up (like any calorie-controlled diet), the controlled periodical fasting of a Fasting Mimicking Diet is of increasing interest to researchers investigating longevity, notably at the Longevity Institute at the University of Southern California. Studies on mice there found that those that fasted were much more responsive to blood-sugar regulating insulin (lack of responsiveness is connected to heart failure, diabetes and obesity) than those on a constantly controlled diet. They lived longer and had about half the rate of age-related diseases, such as cancer and diabetes. They improved cognitively, and the level of inflammation and bone-density loss also slowed.

How does it work? Fasting in this way seems to reduce levels of an insulin-like hormone, growth factor-1, and this makes the body age more slowly and increases the number of regenerative stem cells in different organs. It may boost cell defences against damage and speed up the removal of damaged molecules (researchers postulate that this includes cells linked with neurodegenerative conditions). In a human trial, within three months there was a reduction in markers for heart disease, cancer and diabetes, regardless of what people ate for the rest of the month.

TIP: We mini-fast every day if we finish eating at 7pm and don't eat again till 8am or so. The fasting state kicks in around eight hours after a meal, once the gut has absorbed all the nutrients in food.

What is a Fasting Mimicking Diet?

It replicates the claimed beneficial effects of fasting without putting the body under the stress of actually doing it – fasting can break down muscle to provide the protein we need for energy, which is not useful when we're losing muscle anyway. Also, fasting feels so depleting that most people don't keep it up. Under the Fasting Mimicking regime you eat around a third to a half of the usual daily calories (700–1,100) for five days a month for three months. This diet is low in protein, sugar and carbohydrates and high in healthy fats (nuts, olives), comprising twice-daily vegetable soups, herbal teas and high-nutrient energy bars, plus supplements. Unlike other forms of fasting or calorie-restriction diets, such as the 5:2 diet, it seems relatively easy to keep up – 75 per cent of people completed the first trial. The healthier you are, the less often you need to complete this fast, say its developers; the more risk factors you have and the more obese, the more benefits. Other gerontologists advise that a regular healthy diet (think Mediterranean) may be easier to keep up and less stressful for those with chronic diseases, and that we should be wary of diets that radically change the way we eat.

Warning: Always get a doctor's approval before fasting; it's best to be supervised as you fast.

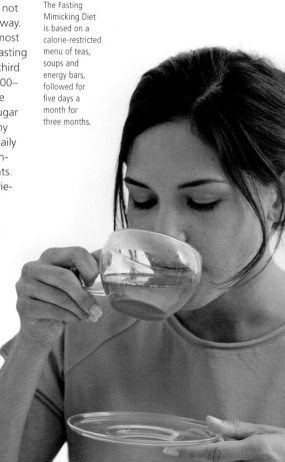

BELOW:
The Fasting Mimicking Diet is based on a calorie-restricted menu of teas, soups and energy bars, followed for five days a month for three months.

Maintaining an appetite

As we head toward our later years we may feel less urge to eat. Our declining sensitivity to taste and smell makes foods seem less appetizing – about a quarter of people over 65 have a reduced ability to detect at least one of the basic tastes (sweet, sour, salty, bitter). Half of us can't detect blends of foods in blind testing.

When we don't eat enough, we risk missing out on vital nutrients that fight the diseases of ageing and make longevity more likely.

We not only feel less hungry as we age, we have less of what we need to take advantage of the nutrients in foods – we experience a reduction in the flow of saliva that starts the digestive process and a decline in gastric acid to break down food. We need fewer calories as we age, due to decreased activity and reduced muscle mass, so we can find ourselves eating meals that

are calorifically adequate and fill us up, but are insufficient in nutrients. Fibre-rich foods especially fill us up without supplying all the nutrients we need. The result is a correlation between increasing age and poor nutritional status.

Under-nutrition contributes to both ill-health and our ability to fight infection and recover from injury. It damages the gut, which is then less able to absorb nutrients, leading to reduced immunity as well as appetite. Weight loss and anorexia are common in older people and often go unrecognized – doesn't everyone

"An excellent thing, the onion, and highly suitable for old people and those with cold temperaments, owing to its nature, which is hot in the highest degree…"

**THE FOUR SEASONS OF THE HOUSE OF CERRUTI,
14TH-CENTURY MANUSCRIPT**

LONGEVITY FOOD

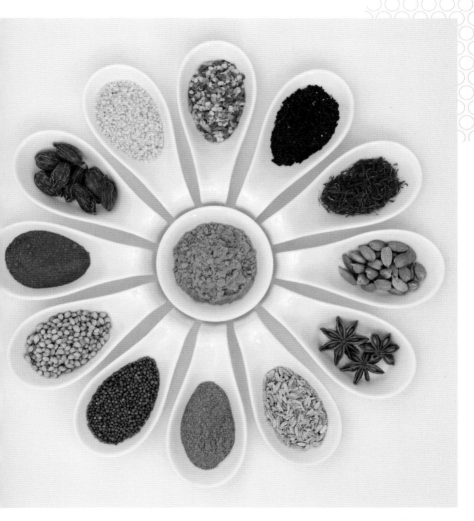

ABOVE: Spices are an easy way to fire up the taste, colour and nutrient content of food to tempt a jaded palate.

NUTRIENT-DENSE FOODS

These ingredients pack a lot of nutrients into a small package, are high in flavour (or absorb flavours well), are low in "fillers" and easily absorbed.

- Eggs
- Fish
- Lean meat
- Liver
- Tofu
- Nuts and seeds

- Whole grains
- Herbs and spices
- Fruit and vegetables
- Seaweed
- Shellfish
- Cocoa

expect an old person to look thin and frail? Symptoms are masked because they echo those of other common age-related diseases. Being depressed when older is also linked with weight loss (it's weight gain in younger adults).

What can we do about this? We need as many nutrients as we can get to counter age-related physiological changes, and the health conditions that may follow, so it's important to keep the diet wide and varied. Eat a little of lots of different foods spread out in several small meals a day, up to five or six if that suits you. You can always snack on highly nutritious items, such as nuts and seeds, in between.

Appetite stimulants and treats can be welcome, maybe some highly flavoured foods for palates that might not be as sensory-charged as they once were. Spice things up with lemon juice and fresh herbs, pepper and mustard, vinegars and seed mixes, and be wary of adding more salt for flavour. Onion stimulates the gastric juices with its fiery mouth-attack, while yogurt is recommended by the WHO for nutritional recovery. And drink plenty of water, too.

TIP: Being more active can raise the appetite – 30 minutes of activity each day is beneficial.

APÉRITIF TIME

Reduced stomach acid can lead to inadequate absorption of nutrients in older people, so you might like to try an apéritif 30 minutes before eating. Apero-hour is common in the western Mediterranean, where longevity seems to follow from a traditional lifestyle. The bitter aromatic herbs in traditional apéritifs, such as Campari or Aperol (and their less traditional non-alcoholic versions), seem to benefit the digestive process. Ingredients such as gentian, angelica or thistle stimulate the mouth to produce saliva, the pancreas to secrete enzymes, and the liver to create bile, aiding digestion.

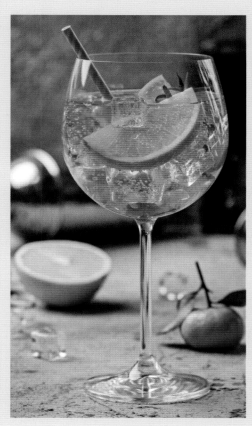

RIGHT: The word "apéritif" derives from the Latin *aperire*, to open: these drinks were thought to open the stomach. Studies show that drinking alcohol just before a meal increases food consumption, but not why.

To supplement — or not

Supplements contain larger doses of nutrients and plant compounds than found in foods alone, and many people choose to take them to fight the effects of ageing and conditions such as cancer and cardiovascular disease.

The UK's Food Standards Agency (FSA) says people over 55 are the main shoppers for supplements. A 2006 study in the US found that by the age of 51, 48 per cent of women and up to 43 per cent of men were taking multivitamins. In the UK, according to an NHS report, 36 per cent of supplement sales in 2009 were for joint-health products. Nutritionists and doctors often argue that eating a wide variety of nutrient-packed foods daily delivers the health benefits we're looking for in a more effective, safe and holistic way.

In many trials, patients don't show the benefits from taking supplements that they do from imbibing the same micro-nutrients in foods. Studies suggest that when the active ingredients of "superfoods", say antioxidants, are separated out and taken as supplements, they may even start to damage the body. Separating out single nutrients wipes out the synergistic reactions that take place when plant ingredients are combined.

Super-strength isn't necessarily super-good for health. If supplements are water-soluble (vitamins C and B), we eliminate the excess in our urine. If they dissolve in fat (vitamins A, D, E and K), they can accumulate in body tissue and liver in concerning amounts. Taking very high doses of *anti*-oxidant supplements (vitamins E, A, betacarotene and C) worries some researchers, who say they may turn into damaging *pro*-oxidants that promote the formation of free radicals, which are said to age us and interfere with the body's defence-mechanism. Calcium supplements have been linked to increased risk of heart disease; vitamin A

TIP: It's tricky to find reliable information about supplements; in the EU, health claims are not allowed on products, while US law doesn't regulate or require evidence to back up the claims on labels or adverts.

RIGHT: Supplements — whether of vitamins, minerals, herbs or plants — should not be considered a substitute for food, says the World Cancer Research Fund.

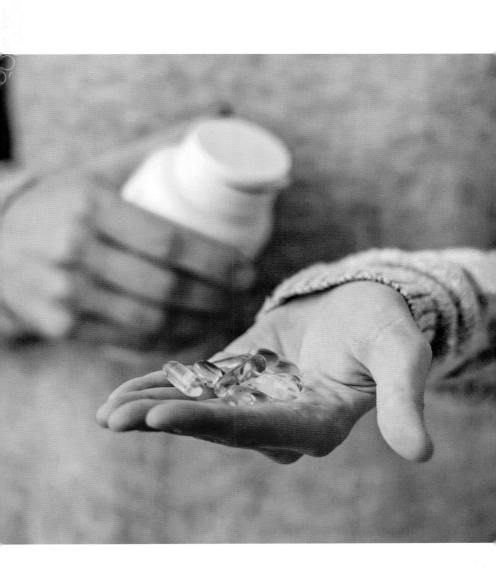

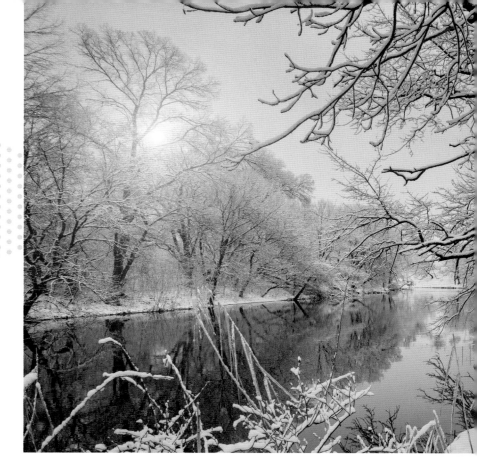

supplements (and a diet high in liver) to increased risk of hip fractures and prostate cancer. A 2010 meta-analysis suggested vitamin E supplements increase mortality through all causes.

There's more. Large randomized trials into multivitamin and mineral supplements over two decades concluded that for the majority of the population they are ineffective and may be deleterious to health. The Cochrane Database of Systematic Reviews (aka the Cochrane Library) undertook an extensive review of supplement

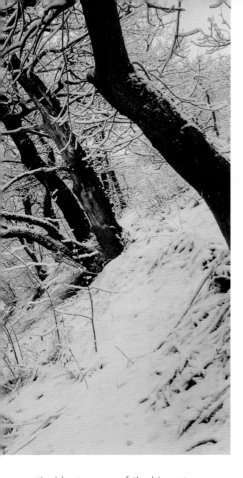

LEFT: During the short winter days, you may want to take a vitamin D supplement – this compensates for lack of sunlight on the skin (which stimulates us to make vitamin D).

That said, some nutritional supplements are recommended if you find it hard to get enough nutrients from food, and we should all take vitamin D, especially in the darker months. Talk to your doctor or a registered dietitian to work out which supplements you need, especially if you're on medication. If your iron is low or you lack energy, see your doctor to have it investigated before taking iron supplements.

Vitamin D
The one supplement we all need. Take 10mcg daily in the winter to maintain optimum bone health (see page 191). Don't take more than 25mcg.

Vitamin E
One research study found that women taking vitamin E experienced one less hot flush a day, but it was a small study, and the US Office of Dietary Supplement has associated supplement-level doses of vitamin E with increased risk of bleeding, and of bleeding in the brain. It can interact with blood-thinning medication.

antioxidants – one of the biggest ever reviews of their effect on mortality. It found no reduction in deaths, but found that taking A, E and betacarotene can increase the risk of dying. Take-out message: supplements are no substitute for food.

Fish oils

If you don't eat fish and have coronary heart disease, the American Heart Association recommends taking 1,000mg of the omega-3 fatty acids DHA and EPA daily and says this dosage may also be useful for people with high blood pressure or cholesterol and diabetes. Consult your doctor before taking, since these supplements can interfere with some medication, including blood-thinners. Avoid fish-liver oil, which contains unsafe levels of vitamin A and can have an adverse effect on bone health.

GLUCOSAMINE

This is the most popular supplement among older people, taken to benefit the health of joints and ease symptoms of osteoarthritis. It's often combined in "neutraceutical" products with chondroitin, both usually extracted from shellfish. The aim is to help rebuild the strength and flexibility of cartilage in the joints. A systematic review published in the *British Medical Journal* found no evidence for the efficacy of either substance, either taken singly or together, although early research points to possible mild pain reduction in some people from taking glucosamine sulfate (1,500mg daily). The supplement is thought safe, but talk to your doctor before taking it, especially if you have asthma. Note that it can interfere with blood-thinning medication; and stop taking it at least two weeks before surgery.

> "Let food be thy medicine and medicine be thy food."
>
> **HIPPOCRATES (ATTRIBUTED)**

RIGHT: We all know milk is a good source of calcium, but so are hard cheeses, dried figs, almonds and sesame seeds. Fish containing edible bones are the most valuable.

LONGEVITY FOOD

238

Calcium

If you're at risk of osteoporosis, over the age of 50 or your diet doesn't provide enough calcium, you might take 800–1200mg a day. This seems to reduce the likelihood of fracture and protect bone mineral density in the femur, neck and lumbar spine.

B12

It gets more difficult to absorb B12 as we get older, so you might consider taking a supplement. Also, since it's not found in fruit, vegetables or grains, you might also consider taking one if you are vegan/vegetarian, and if you don't make enough stomach acid. Take 2mg or less daily.

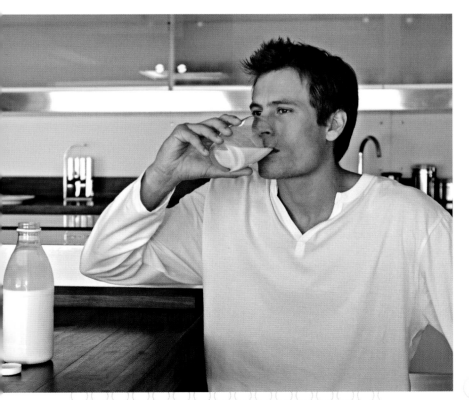

Herbal support

Much less research has been done into herbal remedies as a support for ageing than into nutritional supplements, and any studies tend to be smaller.

Many women turn to natural approaches to help with menopausal symptoms, and red clover, black cohosh, evening primrose oil and other herbal remedies have been studied for the potential relief they can bring. Yet no clear evidence suggests that either herbs or plant oestrogens are effective or safe to take long-term.

The quality of supplements varies hugely between brands, and it's not fully understood how the various compounds in herbs produce their effect. As with nutritional supplements, herbal remedies generally don't have enough good research evidence to convince the national health bodies that approve and monitor the safety and efficacy of prescription or over-the-counter drugs to recommend them – NICE (the National Institute for Health and Care Excellence) in the UK or the FDA (Food and Drug Administration) in the US.

In contrast, mindfulness, hypotherapy and yoga have all shown promising results in combating menopausal symptoms (see page 100). Regular exercise can help relieve hot flushes and increase feelings of wellbeing, while cutting back on caffeine reduces hot flushes and night sweats.

Phytoestrogen supplements

Plant substances called isoflavones are similar in structure to the hormone oestrogen. There are many claims that they relieve menopausal symptoms, but test results, while finding them safe to use in the short term with no increase in adverse effects, aren't consistent. Soy isoflavone supplements seem to be the most beneficial for menopausal symptoms, says the Royal College of Obstetricians and Gynaecologists (a professional association based in the UK), but take only if your periods have

TIP: Look for herbal remedies with the THR (Traditional Herbal Registration) number and logo. This means they meet safely, quality and efficacy standards set by the internationally recognized EU Medicines and Healthcare Regulatory Authority and contain safe-use instructions based on traditional usage.

stopped; taken long-term, they may affect the womb. There's also no convincing evidence that "bioidentical" hormones either relieve symptoms or are safer than conventional Hormone Replacement Therapy (HRT).

It's often suggested that eating more plant foods with mild oestrogenic qualities is a more natural way of easing symptoms – these include chickpeas, lentils, beansprouts, peas and beans, peanuts, sweet potatoes and fermented soy products (tempeh, miso) – but there's no consensus on how much to eat or how often. If you (or your family) have a history of cardiovascular or blood-clotting events or hormone-sensitive cancers (such as breast or ovarian) or if you take anticoagulant medication, it might be best to avoid soy-based products.

Red clover (*Trifolium pratense*)
This legume, which contains isoflavone phytoestrogens, is often recommended to combat symptoms of menopause, and also to lower cholesterol and protect against osteoporosis. It may help reduce hot flushes and night sweats, but research hasn't found clear evidence of efficacy and concludes that it doesn't seem to relieve menopausal symptoms.

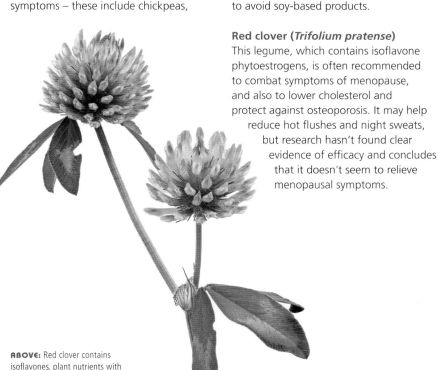

ABOVE: Red clover contains isoflavones, plant nutrients with a similar effect to oestrogen.

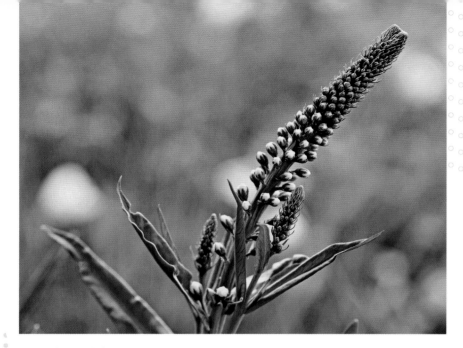

ABOVE: Black cohosh, from the North American herbal tradition, is associated with the relief of menopausal symptoms, but research has not shown how it works.

Flaxseed (*Linum usitatissimum*)

This contains a high concentration of the omega-3 fatty acid ALA. The seed (not the oil) contains phytoestrogens (lignans) and fibre. A number of studies have looked into its effects on menopausal symptoms, and a small study found it worked as well as HRT for mild symptoms; larger studies suggest it doesn't improve symptoms, or protect against bone loss. It may help to lower very high levels of blood cholesterol and lower the risk of breast cancer in postmenopausal women.

Black cohosh (*Actaea racemosa/ Cimicifuga racemosa*)

This is the most-researched herb for menopausal relief – studied since the 1950s – and most often used for reducing hot flushes and night sweats. However, a Cochrane Library review of 16 trials in 2012 concluded there was "overall insufficient evidence" either to support or oppose the use of black cohosh for relieving menopausal symptoms and there are concerns about adverse effects on the liver.

Evening primrose oil (*Oenothera biennis*)

This contains the fatty acid gamma-linolenic acid (GLA) and is used to counter menopausal symptoms. Again, there's no good evidence to back up its use for any health condition, and studies suggest it doesn't work for hot flushes. It can interfere with blood-thinning medication.

Chasteberry (*Agnus castus*)

Long used for reproductive disorders, chasteberry is often recommended to ease menopausal symptoms, but there are very few studies on its efficacy in general and no evidence that it works. Avoid it if you're taking HRT or have a hormone-sensitive condition, including breast cancer.

Dong quai (*Angelica sinensis*)

In Traditional Chinese Medicine this is the remedy most often recommended for women's health and menopause, but there's little research into the latter and one study showed it not to be effective. Another study found it significantly more effective than a placebo in relieving hot flushes when combined with chamomile. It can interfere with blood-thinning medication and sensitize the skin to sunlight.

St John's wort (*Hypericum perforatum*)

The Royal College of Obstetricians and Gynaecologists states that this herb appears to be effective in treating depression during menopause, but doesn't help hot flushes. It can interfere with other drugs and sensitizes the skin to sunlight.

HOMEOPATHY

Encouraging studies have found homeopathy to be helpful in relieving menopausal symptoms and it's completely safe, says the Royal College of Obstetricians and Gynaecologists. In a study of some 400 women in their mid-50s across eight countries, 90 per cent reported a disappearance or lessening of symptoms – particularly a significant reduction in hot flushes by day and night – mostly within 15 days of starting to take a remedy. It's best to visit a homeopath to have your constitutional health assessed and a tailored remedy recommended, but the most commonly prescribed homeopathic remedy for menopausal symptoms is Sepia, which is considered useful for relieving hot flushes, mental confusion, poor circulation, headaches and heavy or painful menstruation. Take 30c daily for short periods while symptoms are intense.

Rosemary for long life

In 2016 a team of US and Italian researchers began a study into the secret of longevity, investigating 300 people in a tiny community in the south of Italy, Acciaroli, above Naples on the Cilento coast. Each participant in the study was over 100 years old, and in the wider community 1 in 60 people were aged over 90 (it's 1 in 163 in the US). As well as this, there was a notable lack of diseases associated with ageing, including Alzheimer's, obesity, heart disease and cataracts. Researchers had already reported on the amazing blood circulation of these people and their low levels of the hormone adrenomedullin (associated with widened blood vessels) – levels similar to people in their 20s and 30s. Researchers also marvelled at the "rampant" sexual activity of these elders.

People here eat a Mediterranean diet – this is rural Italy beside the sea – which means locally caught fish, and chickens and rabbits reared in gardens alongside vegetable and fruit plots.

In fact, this is the area in which the Mediterranean diet was first studied and the term coined in the 1950s. What really intrigues scientists is the huge amount of rosemary in the diet – all the subjects eat it in many different ways. The herb thrives in the ocean climate (it loves moist warmth) and this extra-aromatic wild variety is particularly rich in phytochemicals (such as rosmarinic acid). These have antioxidant, antimicrobial, anti-inflammatory and analgesic properties and are known to stimulate brain function and memory – "that's for remembrance," as Shakespeare wrote.

Since this is mountainous terrain and isolated, it may be that 90-plus years of hill-walking has something to do with the health of the residents. Like many of the other places we've searched for the secret of longevity, this is an isolated place between mountain and sea where the gene pool has probably stayed small. That said, rosemary has been shown to extend the life of fruit flies, mice and worms!

LEFT: Rosemary has long been associated with cognition and memory – in ancient Greece scholars would weave it into their hair to quicken the mind and boost performance.

Tonic herbs

Energy-raising herbs associated with longevity are found in all the traditional pharmacopeias – Ayurvedic, Chinese, European, Native American. They are valued for their healing, rejuvenating and regenerative action and for revitalizing the whole body rather than acting on a single system.

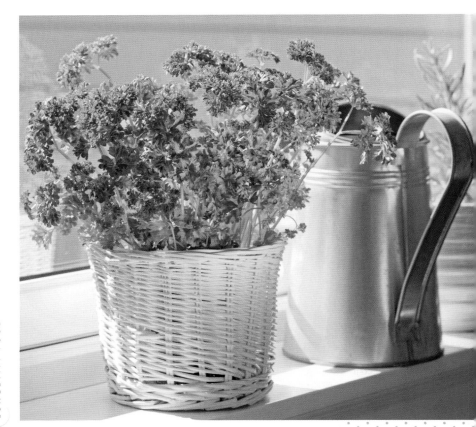

They are said to work by nourishing the body's essence – in the Ayurvedic system, this is known as *ojas*, or life sap, and contributes to the functioning of every tissue. It is especially closely associated with immunity, "coating" the immune system to keep it protected; the sap is said to be analogous to secretions of the pineal gland (see page 339). If this essence is depleted – by over-stimulation, by not eating well, by worry – every part of the body becomes less robust and the immune system weakens, leading to illness. To strengthen *ojas*, specific rebuilding foods (almonds, sesame seeds, honey, warm milk) and herbs are recommended, along with a good amount of rest.

In the Chinese system, this essential vitalizing energy is known as *jing*. Like *ojas*, it's something you are born with and which needs to be nourished in a way that suits your unique constitution. If you keep it consciously kindled, you will live a long and healthy life, it's said; as it becomes depleted, so body and mind start to fade. Symptoms of ageing, such as degeneration of the bones, drying of the skin and weakening of the memory, are associated with a decline in this essential life sap. Herbs that nourish *jing* have a fortifying and moistening action, increasing robustness and enriching every part of the system.

In European herbalism, herbs that strengthen the whole body are known as adaptogens. The term refers to herbs that increase general vitality and boost resistance in stressful or fatiguing situations, physical, mental or emotional. These "non-specific" herbs, which means they work on many systems, are said to nourish, bring body systems into balance and conserve energy as we age. They regulate the adrenal glands and the release of stress hormones, support immunity and have been used traditionally to slow the ageing process. These herbs tend to have a reputation as aphrodisiacs, and have been used by athletes to boost performance and risk-taking.

LEFT: It's simple to raise stimulating herbs on a windowsill; grow from seed or plug plants, rather than supermarket pots, for maximum aroma and bite.

TIP: It's always best to visit a herbalist to be prescribed herbal remedies.

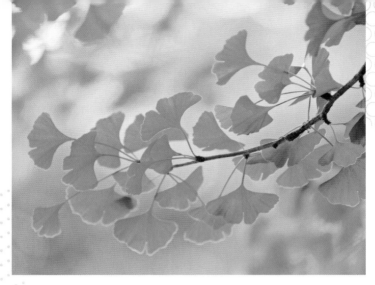

LEFT: Also known as the maidenhair tree, ginkgo is considered a "living fossil" because of its great age (dating from the time of the dinosaurs).

Ginkgo (*Ginkgo biloba*)

Considered the "elixir of youth", this is the go-to remedy for mental decline in older age in the Chinese system – perhaps because of the sympathetic magic of the tree the leaves are taken from, which is one of the oldest living species. Ginkgo seems to act on the circulatory system by dilating blood vessels, reducing the thickness of blood and modifying neurotransmitter signals. It's the top-selling supplement in the UK for memory health. A randomized controlled trial into dementia found it had a small protective effect on dementia caused by damaged blood vessels in the brain, but other studies haven't found robust evidence for its effect on cognitive decline and memory enhancement – nor for its efficacy in lowering blood pressure, preventing heart attack, stroke or age-related macular degeneration. It seems to be safe in moderate amounts, although it can interact with anticoagulant medication; stop taking it at least two weeks before undergoing surgery.

Asian or Chinese ginseng (*Panax ginseng*)

With a history of use dating back more than two thousand years, the ginsenoside components of this plant are valued in China and Korea for replenishing and boosting immune function, increasing stamina and concentration, and relieving problems of ageing in the respiratory, cardiovascular, reproductive and nervous systems. While evidence of the health benefits is inconclusive – there's no real data showing it aids memory and concentration or benefits people with dementia – short-term use seems to be safe, and in a systematic review the Cochrane Library declared that it appeared to have "some beneficial effects on cognition, behavior and quality of life". Products vary when it comes to how much active ingredient they contain (and its quality). Ginseng can interfere with medication and other herbs, and may increase high blood pressure and interfere with hormones. Consult a doctor before taking.

Ashwagandha (*Withania somnifera*)

Referred to as "Indian ginseng", this is a household tonic for ageing in India. With a name that translates as "vitality of the horse", this "ageing-inhibiting" herb is recommended in the Ayurvedic system for its rejuvenative, sedative, nervine and tonic effects, and is given for nervous exhaustion, immune-system problems and complaints of older age, including memory and muscle loss and osteoarthritis. It's considered one of the best tonic herbs to help the body cope with chronic stress, and is used in the Indian healthcare system to treat neurological conditions and support patients in the last stages of cancer. There are no large-scale trials to support its use.

Golden root (*Rhodiola rosea*)

As a longevity tonic, golden root is favoured by Sherpas on Mount Everest to bring the strength and stamina needed to work at altitude. This herb has been used as a performance-enhancer and to treat anxiety, fatigue and stress-related disorders in the mountainous north of the world, from Siberia to Mongolia to Scandinavia. Small studies have found evidence that it can enhance physical performance, relieve mental fatigue and reduce symptoms of depression, but a systemic review found that no two studies reported the same outcomes.

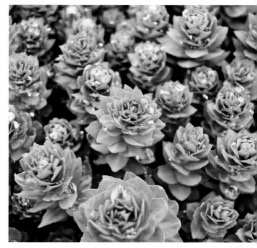

ABOVE: *Rhodiola* is valued for reducing the effects of burnout and fatigue, and restoring cognitive function in those who are exhausted.

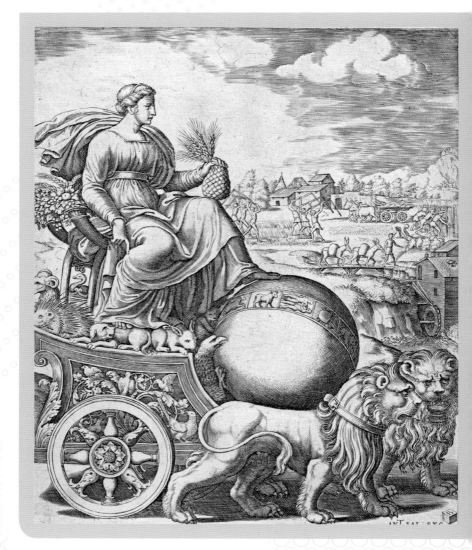

Eternity in a tree

It can feel restorative to contemplate the qualities of ancient plants as we, too, grow older. The oldest tree on the planet has been dated at 9,550 years old, and is in Sweden. The actual tree part looks like a regular Christmas tree – it's a Norway spruce and just 4m (13ft) tall – but its root system is ancient, dating from the end of the last Ice Age. Each trunk survives for 600 years, but the roots keep pushing up new stems over thousands of years.

All the most ancient trees are pines – Bristlecone pines in the White Mountains of California, Huon pines in Tasmania – and in the Chinese world the pine represents longevity and immortality. The pine tree is a powerful symbol connected with those who are departing this world. Pines are often planted around graves as a sign of renewal and constancy – mushrooms are said to sprout from the trees' roots to provide food for the immortals.

The pine is the tree of new year in the Shinto religion, in the same way as the fir tree of Norse legend sits at the centre of Christmas and new-year rites. In the Roman world, too, the pine was an emblem of rebirth and beloved of the goddess Cybele. She ensures the everlasting fruitfulness of the earth as she roams the world in a chariot, carrying a pine tree. Her symbol was used to safeguard new growth and ensure the success of the next year's harvest. The evergreen is ever-young – the self-regenerative powers of the spruce mean it can live almost forever.

LEFT: Cybele, great mother goddess of earth, wild things and fertility, depicted in her chariot drawn by lions. She holds a giant pine cone, symbol of regeneration.

Slow eating

Mindful eating becomes important as we get older and need more nutrients per hit. Mindless grazing can mean we feel full before we've got enough of the ingredients we need to live longer and healthier lives.

The most important thing is to commit to it when we eat – to sit down and treat it as a special time, switching away from everything else to focus on the act of eating and the joy of each taste and texture.

Time taken over each mouthful stimulates the release of enzymes that ensure proper digestion – a 2010 Australian study found that those who chewed less were less likely to meet dietary advice on fibre, sugar, fat and salt.

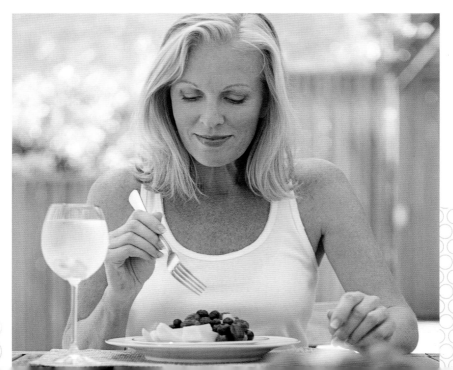

In a 2013 study, mindful eating helped people in mid-life with type-2 diabetes to improve their intake of nutrients, significantly reduce the amount of trans-fats in their diet and improve the amount of fibre eaten. It also helped them control their blood-sugar levels more effectively.

To eat mindfully means being aware, moment-to-moment, of the physical sensations of eating and how they affect our state of mind. It's being aware of when we're physically hungry and acting on it – and being equally aware of psychological hunger and other ways to satisfy it.

A satisfying meal is a sensory meal – it appeals to our human need for colour, texture and scent. A purple-green-yellow plate combining plants with dairy, protein and grain has more appeal than a dish of brown mush, which usually denotes low-value carbohydrates; a meal that combines crunchy and soft, warm and cold keeps the sensory organs piqued, while a mix of old favourites with a few innovative extras keeps the brain engaged.

LEFT: Slow down to eat, giving yourself time to enjoy every mouthful. This aids relaxation and digestion.

ARE YOU WHAT YOU EAT?

A discerning, watching consciousness, if you can cultivate it, is a helpful meditation technique that brings insight and helps us cast off habitual ways of eating that no longer enhance our quality of life. Use these prompts to think about whether your diet serves you, or whether meals have become a habit you might want to rethink:

- Do you eat the same meals you did ten years ago? What about ten years before that?
- Can you remember when certain ingredients or dishes entered your food repertoire? Was it when children were young or work especially busy?
- How are circumstances different now? Have your food choices adapted, too?
- If you choose not to eat some foods, can you explain why? If you stopped eating them a long time ago, can you remember why? Do you feel the same way now?
- Can you express why your favourite dish is your favourite? Is it to do with taste, texture or memories?

Mindfulness on a plate

This exercise awakens awareness of how we eat and is a reminder of the joy of taste and texture. You'll need a table, a chair and a plate of food – and a sense of hunger!

1. Turn off distractions – phone, laptop, TV. Sit at a table on an upright chair with your food in front of you. Sit with your spine upright (a great aid to digestion) and rest your hands on your lap, palms facing up. Bring yourself into the moment by watching your breath moving in and out. Close your eyes.

2. Notice what hungry feels like. Where do you feel the sensations? How would you describe them to someone? Try to avoid clichés – make up your own descriptions.

3. Take your attention to the plate. Look at the food. Keep your hands on your lap for the moment. Notice its colours and arrangement. Pick out the different ingredients and enjoy the way they sit on, or spill over, the plate.

4. Notice the aromas. Can you identify any individual scents? When other thoughts come to mind, let them pass, constantly bringing yourself back to the food on the plate.

5. Now cut and fork or spoon the food. Notice the textures – smooth and rough, tough and tender, oozing and fluid.

6. Close your eyes as you place a small amount in your mouth. Put your cutlery down and rest your hands in your lap again. Pause and notice the flavours activating the taste buds at various points on your tongue. Can you work out where the sensations start and how they move around the mouth?

THE ART OF THE PLATE

Traditionally, in India each meal is considered to be made up of 32 mouthfuls, and the stomach is visualized as having four parts – two for food, one for liquid and one left empty to allow energy to circulate.

7. As you chew, notice the muscles in your jaw and neck working. When do you have to swallow? What makes you do this? Open your eyes and take another mouthful. Does it taste different when you have the visual distraction of your environment?

8. Slow down as you eat, so that you are aware of each mouthful in the moment. After finishing, sit still in silence for a few minutes. Can you visualize the food being taken up in the gut, circulating through your body systems and being transformed into energy?

BELOW: A mix of textures, colours, scents and tastes makes for the most sensory and mindful mealtime.

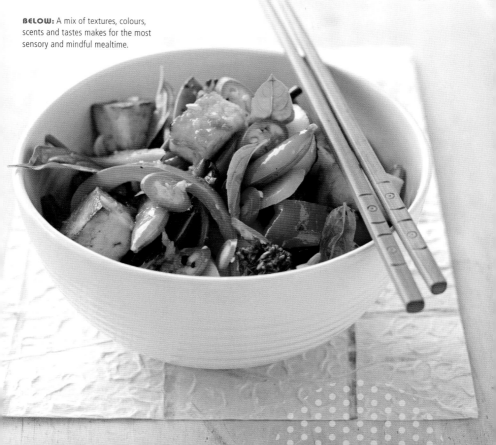

Ayurvedic eating

I n the Indian longevity practice of Ayurveda, a well-functioning digestive system is regarded as one of the most important ways of keeping the body in balance and protecting health. Undigested food is a main cause of all health problems, according to Ayurvedic medicine, which recommends foods and yoga poses (see page 226) to build *agni*, the inner fire that ensures good digestion.

Food that tastes delicious is considered to be the most easily digested and best able to build strength and sensory awareness. Ayurveda classifies foods in terms of six tastes, or *rasa*, linked to the

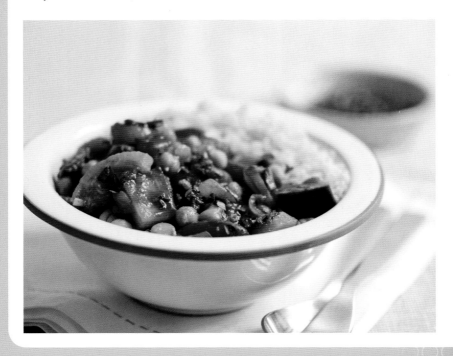

LEFT AND RIGHT: Seasonal eating is a key tenet of the Ayurvedic diet, bringing the body into balance with its environment as well as the season's *dosha*. Spring/summer is a time for pungent, bitter and astringent tastes, while moving into winter, sweet, sour and salty foods are considered most nourishing.

elements water, earth, fire, air, space. Cooking is about blending these tastes in such a way that they "delight" the brain and thus stimulate digestion, releasing optimum nutrients. *Rasa* means both "essence" and "delight", recognizing that food affects emotional wellbeing. The way in which we eat also matters – meal-times should be calm and relaxing, which promotes digestion.

Even though each food is a blend of tastes, one may predominate, and we all need some of each to bring body and emotions into balance, according to our individual constitution or *dosha* (see page 17). In Ayurveda, when everything is balanced, there is no illness and life is long. Eaten in excess, any of the tastes upsets this balance in the body.

Eating right for the season and climate is considered health-giving, too. In winter and damp regions opt for warming, pungent foods and in summer and dry regions cold, dry ones. Sweet tastes are thought to be nourishing in older age, promoting strength and long life, while sour tastes stimulate saliva and appetite, and pungency boosts digestion.

THE SIX TASTES IN AYURVEDA

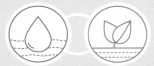

- **Sweet (water + earth)**
  Sugary, starchy foods including grains and dairy. These are grounding, strengthening for the body, and nurture contentment

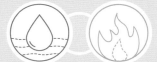

- **Sour (water + fire)**
  Acidic, fermented foods, such as lemons and vinegar. These kick-start the appetite and the digestion and awaken the senses

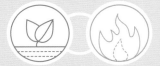

- **Salty (earth + fire)**
  Alkaline, salty foods, such as seaweed and olives. These boost mineral absorption and calm the nerves

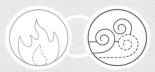

- **Pungent (fire + air)**
  Spicy, piquant foods, such as onions and ginger. These act as digestive and circulatory stimulants, and quicken the mind

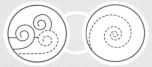

- **Bitter (air + space)**
  Cooling and tannic foods, including green vegetables, herbs and teas. These promote elimination and bring about a sense of clarity

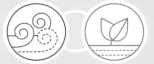

- **Astringent (air + earth)**
  Dry, light foods, such as beans and sprouted foods. These have a cooling effect and boost firmness of mind

COOLING FOODS FOR HOT FLUSHES

Ayurvedic practitioners advise that eating to rebalance your constitution, or *dosha*, brings best results, but these foods are recommended more generally to cool *pitta*, or inner fire:

Eat more
• sweet, bitter and astringent foods
• rice, milk
• vegetables and juicy fruit
• digestive spices, such as fennel and cardamom

Eat fewer
• salty, sour foods
• foods preserved in vinegar
• hot spices, such as chillies, pepper and mustard

BELOW: Spices that aid digestion, such as cardamom, may be recommended during menopause by Ayurvedic practitioners.

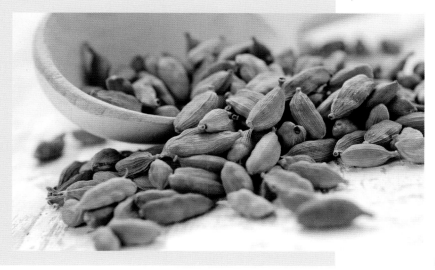

Okinawa: land of immortals

The most extreme version of the traditional Japanese diet is found on the Pacific Ocean islands of Okinawa prefecture, or the Ryukyu Islands, 640 km (400 miles) south of Japan. The diet includes seven portions of vegetables daily and two of soy, fish three times a week and seafood, plus whole grains, legumes and daily fermented foods. Hardly any dairy is eaten and only a little meat or eggs, although pork is the main feature of feasts. The people who eat this traditional diet have a lowered risk of all the major age-related diseases – cardiovascular, dementia, diabetes, and hormone-sensitive cancers, such as breast and prostate. The people of Japan have traditionally had exceptionally long life expectancy; the people of Okinawa have the highest life expectancy on the planet. The UN says they have the highest proportion of centenarians in the world.

Is it all to do with diet? Might lifestyle play a role? The tradition of stopping to eat and sharing food with friends is alive on these islands, as is the motto *Hara Hachi Bu* – stop eating when 80 per cent full. People commit to share work, including food preparation, as a community and gather in social groups (Moai). Meditation and the martial arts are common practices, and an indigenous belief system honours the ancestors and spirits of place. Women keep alive this spiritual and socially connected way of life, organizing rituals and acting as mediums with the spirit world – they are also the longest-lived. Then there's the idea that life is lived backward, so that as we age we get younger, eventually returning in death to the womb.

Like many regions that have an unusual number of centenarians, this is a fiercely independent place and much fought-over. The elderly – and their ancestors – have lived through periods of near-starvation. In World War Two, this was the site of the bloodiest conflict in the Pacific War; around a third of the native population were slaughtered. More people died here than in Hiroshima and Nagasaki when they were bombed. We know that periods of calorie-restriction prime us to live longer. And might there be some urge for redemption in our searches for the source of eternal life in beautiful places we've destroyed through war?

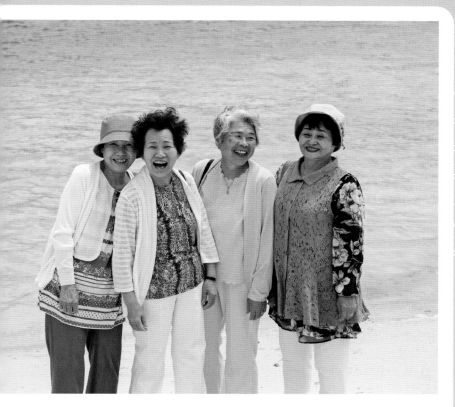

What we do know is that when the Okinawans began eating like the rest of us – more rice and bread, milk for the first time – the incidence of cancers doubled. Healthy habits that were developed pre-1940 may die with the current generation of elders.

ABOVE: The islands of subtropical Okinawa, Japan, have been home to some of the longest-lived people to be found on the planet.

Part 3

LONGEVITY MIND:
relaxed, conscious, sharp

No one really knows how the mind works, but we do know the brain changes with age and, you guessed it, declines in function. In fact, it shrinks physically – some 5 per cent per decade after the age of 40, speeding up post-70 – and the loss of volume is linked with a loss of neuropsychological function. Reduced flow of blood to the brain and blood-pressure problems also contribute. The prefrontal cortex is the area most affected – the part of the brain associated with executive function, the ability to manage such things as reasoning, problem-solving, planning and decision-making. It orchestrates the rest of the brain to set us working toward goals and directs our focus. It also moderates our behaviour and emotional reactions, ensuring we behave by society's rules, and seems to be connected with feelings of guilt and remorse when we fail.

Neurotransmitters carrying messages between neurons also decline with age. We lose a major one of these, dopamine, at 10 per cent per decade through adulthood, and this correlates with shrinking cognition and motor skills. Fading levels of another neurotransmitter, serotonin, affect plasticity, the ability of the brain to change. Declining sex hormones, especially in women, seem to be linked to memory problems, and lowered growth-hormone levels may affect the function of the hippocampus, the part of the brain that processes and stores memories and regulates emotion.

All this means the brain slows with age – we might first notice that we're less able to process information quickly, or that we're more easily distracted, unable to tune out and concentrate or divide attention effectively between tasks. It becomes harder to juggle information and to conceptualize a problem, make a decision, act on it and change tack as circumstances change. Our mental function and memory skills are most acute in our 20s, levelling off in our 50s and 60s. We tend to notice changes from around 65, and there's a sharp drop in mental powers in the years leading up to death.

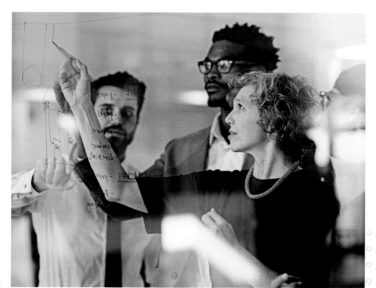

LEFT: Continuing education is one of the most useful things we can do to keep the memory sharp and the brain working at its best.

RIGHT: A comparison between the brain of a 22-year-old man (top row) and that of a 96-year-old woman (bottom row): brain shrinkage shows in the extensive white areas.

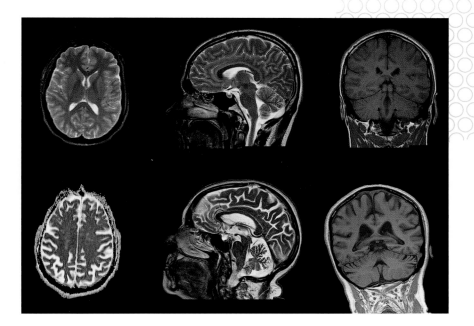

TIP: Every brain ages at a different rate. To find your current mental age, search online for My Mental Age Test and take the test.

Now for some good news – we can reverse some of the decline in function, and the brain adapts, compensating by switching on different areas and creating new neural pathways and "scaffolding" to keep us sharp. Eating well helps – risk of cognitive decline is increased by a high-calorie, low-antioxidant diet. Periods of fasting seem to protect against mental decline, as does increasing the amount of fish and seafood we eat. Moderate to low amounts of alcohol may stimulate the hippocampus.

Regular exercise helps hugely by promoting cerebral blood flow and stimulating the growth of brain cells; also perhaps by stabilizing blood-sugar – spikes may affect the memory-formation area of the brain. Increased fitness reduces age-related declines in function, and the lower your risk of cardiovascular disease, the lower the biological age of your brain.

LONGEVITY MIND

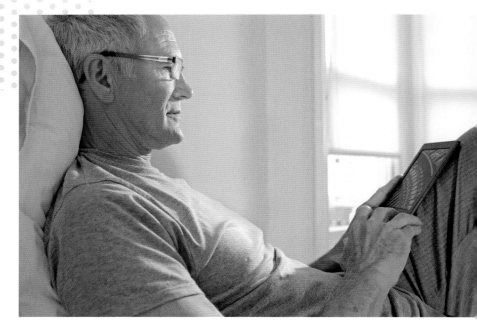

YOUTHFUL BRAIN FORMULA

- Frequent exercise
- A diet that benefits the cardiovascular system
- Regular mental workouts
- Calmness in the face of stress
- An active social life

Active people who eat a healthy diet are more likely to score well on cognitive tests than inactive people of a similar age or younger. That's not solely due to cardio-training, either. Activities that promote balance and coordination (see page 44) improve cognitive ability, too. A 21-year study led by the Albert Einstein College of Medicine in New York found that people who danced frequently had a 76 per cent lower incidence of dementia – a higher reduction than in people who did intellectual brain training.

"An old person has eaten wisdom."

AFRICAN PROVERB

IN WITH THE NEW

Although we might not be able to stop time, we can change how time feels by exposing ourselves to new experiences. Have you noticed how the first few days of a holiday seem to last forever? That's because the brain is firing off in reaction to all the novelty. The stimulation of new places, people, food and language lays down lots of memories, so when we look back, all that extra texture lengthens our perception of time.

The most consistently helpful thing we can do for the brain, though, seems to be continuing education – the more educated we are, the better the reserves we build in the early years to protect ourselves from brain-ageing in later decades. A university degree seems to slow ageing by up to ten years, until age 75. It also protects against dementia and is associated with a longer life. No college degree? We can more than make up for it with continual brain stimulation from an intellectually demanding job or pastime. Exercising the brain with word or number puzzles, by reading and by engaging with ideas helps train the memory and intelligence so well that in tests we can perform as well as younger people.

The best news is that some cognitive skills grow with age. Extra decades of experience make us better at the kind of higher-order reasoning that involves weighing up facts and estimating based on past example. As older people, we're better at coming at problems from different perspectives and bringing morals to bear on a subject.

Ancient wisdom

This wisdom, known as crystallized intelligence, is different from knowledge. Unlike memory, reasoning and processing speed, it stays the same or even increases with age. Acquired through experience, it is characterized by compassion and tolerance, and an awareness of multiple perspectives and uncertainty. The Greek philosopher Plutarch posed the question: *Whether an*

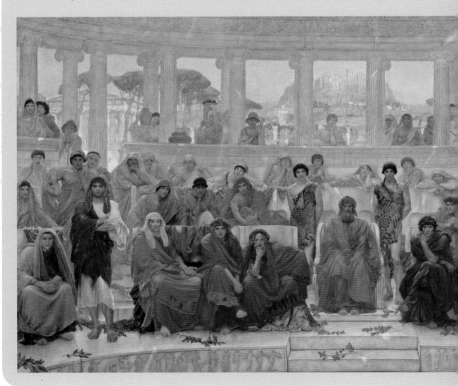

Old Man Should Engage in Public Affairs? In his treatise of the same name he answers yes! While young people bring youthful bodies to the affairs of state, seniors offer "sapience profound", which he explains as reason, judgment, frankness and the "beauties of the soul", that is justice, moderation and wisdom. And since these mature into their "proper quality late and slowly", he says it's madness if older people are let go from leadership roles. Age, he says, only "increases our power for leading and governing".

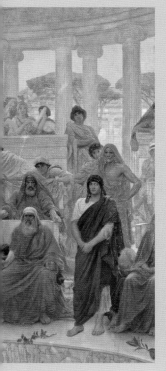

The words "senior" and "senator" share a Latin root, *senatus*, which means an "assembly of elders". So, calling someone "senile" is actually respectful. The Greek words for great age, *gera*, *geron*, also refer to privilege and the rights of the position held by those elected to councils of elders, *gerusia*. The wisdom of the old is necessary to society. It is in the old that traditions are preserved and passed on – knowledge of a society's rites and myths, customs and ceremony, and the choice about when and how (and if) to pass that on confers huge authority. Memory is power, and those with the most are regarded as magical in many cultures, closer to the ancestors and equipped to mediate between past lives and future worlds.

LEFT: In *An Audience in Athens During Agamemnon by Aeschylus*, a 19th-century painting by William Blake Richmond, a mature figure of seniority and authority dominates the centre of the canvas. He is a priest of Dionysus, god of theatre and fruitfulness.

Stress and ageing

Stress is known to affect the ageing brain and to be an important risk factor for cognitive decline. It seems likely that the more stressful life events we live through, the worse our cognitive function as we age – in studies, it correlated with worse performance on cognitive tasks. When we're older, Less stress equals cognitive performance on a par with younger people.

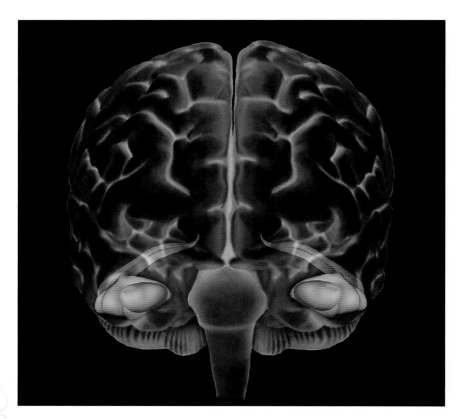

We all need a shot of adrenaline and cortisol (stress hormones) to get things done – if we had no sense of urgency or heightened reflexes, we'd never meet deadlines or manage to cross the road safely. Stress hormones are released in response to a perceived threat. They cause blood pressure to rise, muscle tension to increase, the heart to beat faster and breathing to become more rapid and shallower. All this equips the body to react to the threat by running away or fighting. Whichever action we choose activates the parasympathetic nervous system, so that once the threat has passed, we are automatically switched back from a physical state of preparedness into a relaxed "rest and digest" mode.

Psychological stressors are not as easily dispersed by fighting or fleeing – they're more invasive. Feeling threatened emotionally amplifies the significance of the stressor, and the very process of ruminating on it, letting negative thoughts run away with us, prolongs stress arousal. We risk becoming even more upset by our emotional response and falling into a prolonged state of reactivity. If we don't act to release this tension and it builds up over time, the constantly elevated blood pressure and heart rate, the changes to breathing and blood-sugar levels, the increased inflammation and less responsive immune system that result lead to ill-health and cognitive decline.

In the brain, stress seems to affect the hippocampus, having an effect on short-term memory and our ability to exclude intrusive thoughts, make sound decisions and control impulses. Chronic psychological stress – typically caused by lack of control over living conditions or social environment – is especially toxic for the brain. Like depression, it seems to affect the length of telomeres, the protective cap at the end of chromosomes (see page 14). When a cell divides, its telomeres shorten until they become too eroded, then the chromosomes get damaged. The cell can't reproduce itself and dies. That's ageing. Shortened telomeres have been linked with many conditions associated with ageing, from osteoporosis to heart disease. Telomeres are repaired by the enzyme telomerase, which allows cells to go on dividing, making healthy copies of themselves. Chronic stress promotes the release of cortisol, which suppresses the production of telomerase.

LEFT: The seahorse-shaped hippocampi, picked out here in pink, deep in the temporal lobes, are associated with learning, memory and spatial navigation.

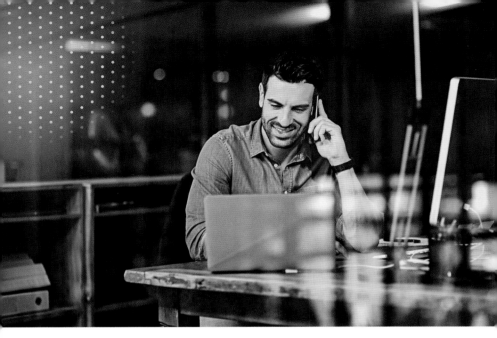

ABOVE: An ability to stay calm and focused amid daily stresses is associated with increased happiness and productivity.

Exercise and a healthy diet are the best buffers against stress, followed by a supportive social network, but changing the way we react to stress is vital, too. Since the 1960s, research studies have shown that meditation and mindfulness reduce mental anxiety and reset habitual stress pathways that build up over time. In short, becoming aware of our thoughts, feeling more in control of how we process them and accepting that emotional experiences don't need to overwhelm us induces a relaxation response that brings stress-hormone levels back to normal, relaxes muscles, slows the heart rate and undoes other damaging physical reactions. In studies, it correlates with increased mental performance, greater satisfaction in work tasks and an improved ability to study and retain information.

If stress physically ages us by damaging the telomeres, then mindful meditation winds back the clock. Breathing-awareness techniques are a great place to start learning mindfulness and meditation, and have long been valued as a longevity practice in themselves.

Meditation for long life

When we become aware of our thoughts moment by moment, and can look at the effect emotions have on us in a non-judgmental way, we feel more in control and able to roll with the inevitable stuff life throws at us as we age.

Then we can more accurately judge what's worth reacting to and how real a perceived threat is. We feel less distressed about being distressed. This buffers us against the negative effects of stress, and that seems to slow the rate at which cells age. Meditation and mindfulness teach us how to do this. Living life in the moment is the only known way to slow time.

Meditation seems to activate the part of the brain that atrophies with age, the prefrontal cortex, and activation of this region correlates with feelings of wellbeing. When we meditate, heart and breathing rates reduce and blood flow to the brain increases. A deep but mentally alert state of rest associated with high alpha brain waves ensues, and scans of the brain show meditation increasing activity in the hippocampus.

Studies of people who do Transcendental Meditation (TM), the most researched form of meditation, show they have a biological age significantly lower than their chronological age, with mental, physical, cognitive and perceptual abilities equivalent to those of much younger people. People who meditate seem to have lower levels of cortisol and levels of DHEA (aka the youth hormone) similar to people five to ten years younger. DHEA decreases with age and low levels correlate with disease and mortality.

Meditation seems helpful in dealing with many diseases associated with ageing. It's useful for reducing high blood pressure – TM was shown to be more effective than either relaxation or regular care regimes at rapidly reducing systolic and diastolic pressure levels for men and women (it seems to keep blood vessels open). Since it has no side-effects and is easy to practise at home, meditation is routinely recommended by doctors to those at risk from stroke. It may also be helpful for heart disease. It can help us live with chronic pain by releasing some of the muscle tension that contributes to the pain cycle. The Benson-Henry Institute in Massachusetts, US, found that in the year after relaxation-response training participants' interactions with healthcare providers dropped by around 43 per cent.

LONGEVITY MIND

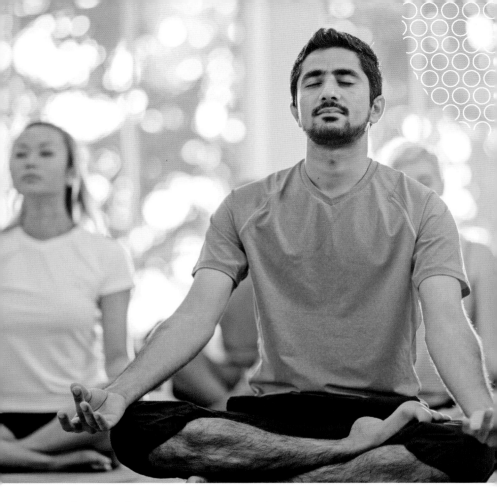

Meditation is often included in complementary programmes to support cancer care and can help reduce unpleasant symptoms that accompany chemotherapy treatment. Some studies have shown that cancer patients who meditated survived for twice as long as those who did not.

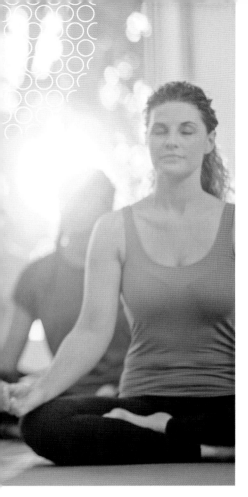

ABOVE: It's most effective to learn
how to meditate from a teacher and
to join a group that sits regularly to
share ideas and concerns.

Mindfulness

The act of non-judgmental, moment-to-moment awareness has been less well studied than meditation until recently, but numerous studies into mindfulness-based stress relief (MBSR) demonstrate its positive effects. MBSR encompasses silent sitting, walking meditations, body scans and mindful movement, such as yoga, qigong and engaged dance forms such as tango (see page 326), among other activities. Mindfulness seems to trigger an anti-inflammatory action, to boost white blood-cell count and antibody response, and to stimulate the part of the brain that governs immune-suppression. It has been shown to prevent atrophy in the hippocampus and promote neuroplasticity. It may also be helpful in improving menopausal symptoms, including hot flushes.

Mindfulness can be especially easy to fit into a busy life because you don't have to set aside time to do it – we can use the techniques to bring a meditative awareness to every activity, from brushing our teeth to weight-training, simply by staying aware of every action and letting go of intrusive thoughts. We relax and make space for a more enriching mental and sensory life.

Silent sitting

This is the classic position used for meditation. The Zen term *zazen* translates as "just sitting" and refers to a state we achieve when just being, aware of but unfazed by sensation, thought and emotion. It's important that we sit upright when meditating – as yoga guru BKS Iyengar taught, when the spine is upright, the brain is alert. You might like to use a focusing technique, such as breathing or counting, to help bring your mind into the present while sitting (see page 292). Practise for three to five minutes at first, building up to 20 minutes twice a day. You can sit on a chair or cross-legged on the floor with your back supported by a wall, or kneel. What's most important is that your body feels relaxed when you start and your spine is straight.

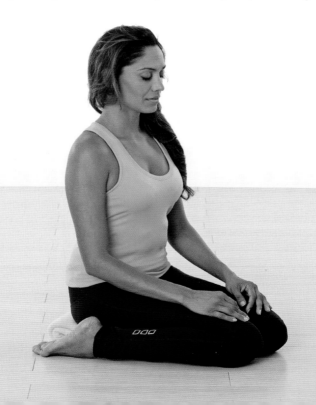

OVERCOME INTRUSIVE THOUGHTS

When you meditate, try to be aware of thoughts the moment they occur. This stops us following them into stories – lovely as they are, stories are engrossing and draw us away from the present moment into plans for the future or retellings of the past. As you practise, your perception of intrusive thoughts will sharpen and you'll be more able to halt a daydream at will and keep your focus more keenly in the now.

1. Sit or kneel comfortably. If you prefer, place a folded blanket beneath your feet and another under your buttocks. Keep your spine erect, and ears and shoulders aligned; look ahead.

2. Rest your hands on your thighs or knees, palms down. Half-close your eyes and focus forward and just down; let your gaze soften. It helps to face a blank wall to avoid visual distraction.

3. Take your focus inside and notice your breath moving in and out through your nostrils. Calmly move into witnessing mode, watching your thoughts, emotions and sensations as if you are a disinterested observer. When a train of thoughts carries you away, as it will, do not chastise yourself; simply acknowledge it, ask it to pass and return to awareness of your breath moving in and out. Check your posture and relax your shoulders.

4. When it's time to finish, become aware of the room around you. Wriggle your fingers and toes, then carefully unfold your legs.

Candle concentration

The candle-gazing meditation *trataka* uses the physical focus of a flame to calm the mind. As you look at the tip of the flame only, your awareness of the flow of ideas through your brain slows and eventually is suspended. This one-pointed or single-focus meditation can be particularly helpful at stressful times, when it's difficult to keep your mind on one thing. You will need a low table and a nightlight.

1. Sit comfortably upright, hands resting on your knees or thighs. Place a nightlight level with your eyes.

2. Settle yourself by watching your breath moving in and out, then focus your gaze on the tip of the flame, at the point at which its form and colour disappear.

3. Keep your gaze steady on the flame for up to 30 seconds, trying not to blink. Then close your eyes and visualize the flame in your mind's eye. Feel as if it is cleansing your mind, burning off thoughts and turning them into vapour.

4. When the image has faded, open your eyes and repeat the gaze. As thoughts intrude, let them burn away and return to the flame. Practise for three minutes, allowing the image of the flame to cleanse your mind of distraction.

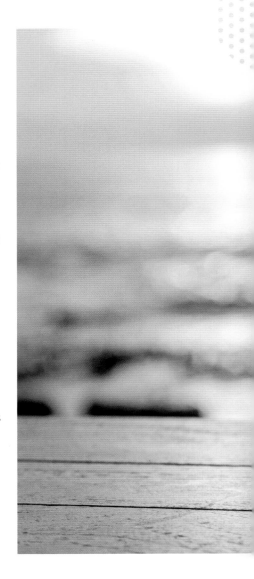

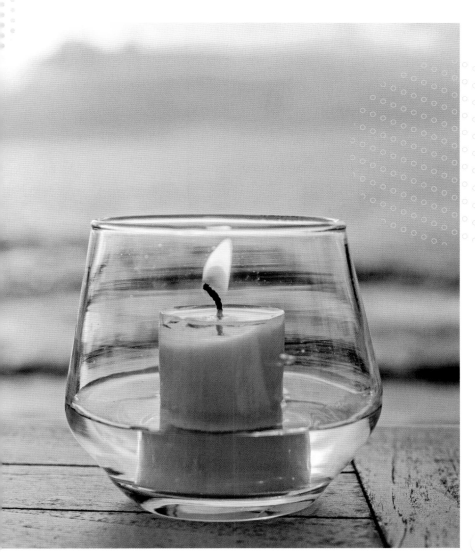

Mindful walking

This is a really accessible way to sample mindfulness. It's good for settling the mind before seated meditation, and effective when you want to keep meditating but your legs and feet have fallen asleep. You will need enough space to take about 30 paces in a straight line. Have bare feet if possible.

1. Stand at the start of your walking track. Look forward and lift your upper body, feeling your spine and neck lengthen. Let your arms hang loosely by your sides, shoulders relaxed. Centre yourself by closing your eyes and watching your breath move in and out.

2. Open your eyes and look down and slightly forward, softening and broadening your gaze – imagine looking out through your temples. On an inhalation, shift your right foot forward. Exhale. On the next inhalation, step your left foot forward.

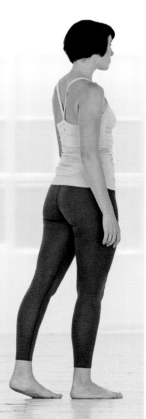
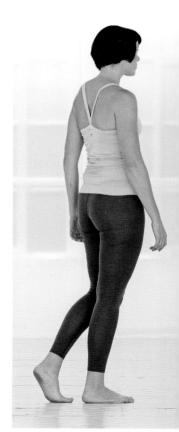

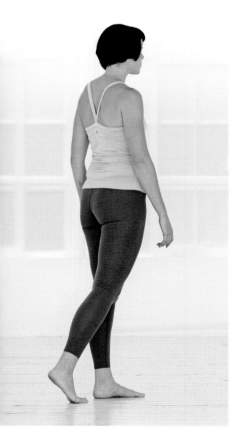

3. Continue along your path at this slow pace. Notice your weight transferring from heel to toe with each step. Enjoy each heel peeling away from the floor, feel the push through the ball of your foot and the big toe anchoring you.

4. Keeping walking, now noticing how your arms fall into rhythm with your gait. Take your awareness to the back of your body and consciously slow down, if you've been pushing forward with your chest and chin. Notice your abdomen – can you feel the movement starting there?

5. When you reach the end of your track, turn and walk back again. Look gently forward, not at your feet. Stay with each step, aware simply of the repetitious action of each foot lifting, moving forward, lowering to the ground and carrying you. Bring your focus back to this when thoughts wander. Repeat for as long as you like.

Walking into knowledge

A journey on foot has always been linked with a quest for inner peace, calm and connection with something bigger than us, be that the divine, nature or our place in the state of things, and it is often undertaken at times of transition. The Christian pilgrimage along the Camino to Santiago de Compostela in Spain or the Muslim Hajj to Mecca share the notion that as you draw nearer the physical end of the path, you progress further along the journey toward self-discovery, transformation or a new phase of life.

The mythologist Joseph Campbell built on Jungian archetypes and popularized the idea of the hero's journey. The hero (or heroine) archetype is a figure who sets out on a quest – to find the holy grail or the golden fleece, to kill the monster. The journey is arduous, physically and emotionally, and the hero has to overcome a series of trials, which increase in intensity as the journey goes on. Along the way the hero uncovers a truth about himself and faces a choice – whether to continue as before or to embrace the truth and struggle to overcome it. There is a dark night of the soul, a point toward the end of the journey when all seems lost and the forces of antagonism are at their most intense. If the hero can make the right choice at that moment, he is rewarded, possibly not with what he wanted, the ring, but with what he needs – self-knowledge. A homecoming follows when the hero, finally, at the end of the journey, is able to accomplish what he could not at the beginning.

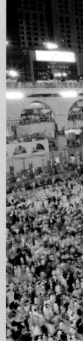

RIGHT: At the annual Hajj pilgrimage, worshippers circle the ancient building of the Kaaba, in the Grand Mosque in Mecca, Saudi Arabia.

The oldest quest story is the *Epic of Gilgamesh*, written some three thousand years ago in Mesopotamia, in which the eponymous hero sets out to discover the secret of eternal life, following the death of his best friend. He must learn through his journey into the wilderness to accept not only his friend's death but his own mortality and to become a good and wise king, which he does – and returns home to rule for 126 years.

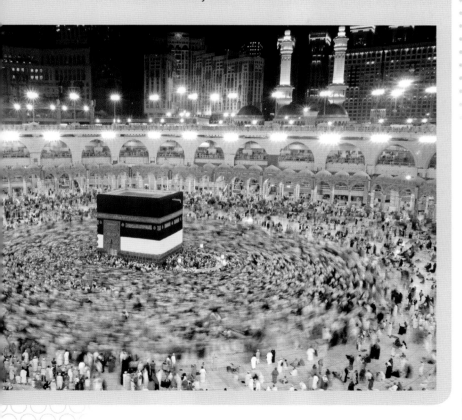

Long, slow breathing

The simplest way to experience mindfulness is to watch the breath. When we do this, we are meditating — it's that easy and it protects against the ageing effects of stress.

Inevitably, as we follow the inflow and exit of air though the nostrils, as we feel the diaphragm move up and down and the ribcage expand, we are witnessing the present moment and excluding everything else from our thoughts.

Emotionally, witnessing the breath shows us how to stand back and watch ourselves in everyday situations until we become aware of our habitual reactions. Such self-awareness can prompt us to stop as we start to anger, and to pick ourselves up kindly on habits that make us feel bad about ourselves. We learn how to temper difficult emotions and harvest good from bad. Physically, deeper breathing turns off the fight-or-flight stress response and activates the parasympathetic nervous system, the rest, recuperate and heal setting.

Better breathing becomes more vital as we age, for oxygen delivery and to rid us of carbon dioxide. Peak lung function is around age 25; after about 35 it starts to decline. As we age we tend to breathe less efficiently — the intercostal muscles around the ribcage and diaphragm become weaker (especially in men), the

RIGHT: Every breath matters — becoming more mindful is as easy as slowing down to tune into each inhalation and each exhalation.

bones of the ribs can thin and the spine can change in shape. Air sacs in the lungs lose their buoyancy from around age 50, leading to dead space. All this makes it more difficult to take a full breath in and to exhale fully — that ability is 20 per cent diminished when we're sedentary (as we tend to be with age). We're at a mechanical disadvantage if we don't practise deep breathing, which helps both to keep the muscles strong and the lungs expanding and contracting effectively.

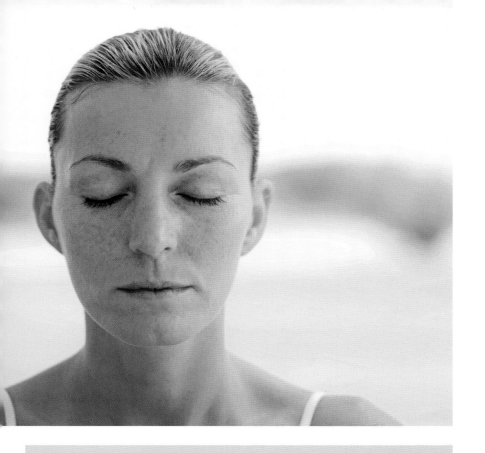

THE MOUSE AND THE TORTOISE

In many traditions, there is the notion that we are born with an allotted number of breaths. Aristotle called it our finite amount of "vital substance". When we have used them up, we die – simple. One example to support this idea cites the mouse and the tortoise. A mouse breathes very fast (90–170 breaths per minute) and lives at most three years; a tortoise breathes slowly (3–4 breaths per minute) and lives up to 400 years.

Breath control

Techniques used to control breathing have long been considered a means to achieve longevity. Practical ways to slow the breath include lengthening the inhalation and thus maximizing the time for oxygen/carbon-dioxide transfer, making exhalation more complete and effective, and strengthening the muscles of the chest.

"For breath is life,
and if you breathe
well you will live
long on earth."

SANSKRIT PROVERB

TIP: Practise yoga twists (see pages 224–5) to build the muscles we use for breathing and release tension that stiffens the ribcage, preventing a full and easy breath.

THE VAGUS NERVE

The vagus or "wandering" nerve is the longest and most complex of the 12 cranial nerves and has the farthest reach, running from the brain down to the abdomen. Its multiple branches reach out to the sense organs of nose, eye, ear and tongue, the muscles of the face and those that control swallowing and speech, the heart, lungs and diaphragm, down to the gastrointestinal tract. The impulses this nerve transmits balance the nervous system – it controls heart and breathing rate, blood pressure and digestion, and can decrease inflammation and dissolve the effects of stress and fear.

When its "tone" is high, we feel well and the body systems function effectively. Lowered tone is linked with many of the common conditions of ageing, from heart attack and stroke to depression, digestive disorders and rheumatoid arthritis. Stimulation of the nerve (by electronic impulses delivered through an implant in the chest) is used to regulate mood and reduce depression, lower risk of heart disease and treat inflammation and memory disorders and Alzheimer's.

Deep diaphragmatic breathing with a focus on the out-breath can activate the vagus nerve, and may account for the ability of yoga breathing techniques to turn on the parasympathetic nervous system, or rest-and-digest response. Ear acupuncture is also used to stimulate this nerve.

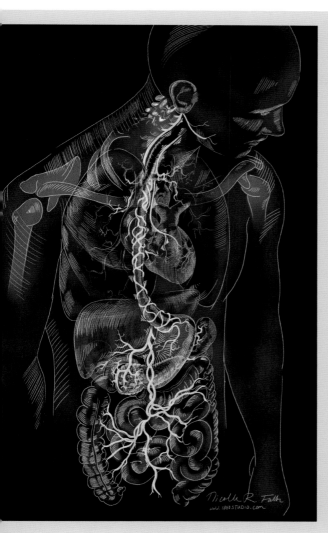

LEFT: The multiple branches of the vagus nerve wander from the brain down into the intestines: of all the body's nerves, this has the widest distribution.

The tortoise

The world's oldest terrestrial animal, thought to be 183 years old, is a tortoise living on the island of St Helena. Our longest living vertebrate species, the tortoise is considered a symbol of longevity in China and Japan, its form replicated in amulets worn as protection from disease and other forces of malevolence. In the yoga tradition, the tortoise is admired for its ability to draw in its senses and withdraw from the stress of the world, to look inside and gather up life-sustaining energy and strength.

In stories, the tortoise is valued for its patience and endurance. Its slow, unflappable nature powers it to the finishing line before the excitable and distracted hare. The form of a tortoise appears as an architectural feature, solidly supporting buildings and columns, just as in Indian mythology it is a turtle's legs that support the mythical elephant that holds up the world. The domed shell stands for the curve of the earth, and in many traditions the tortoise links the life of this world with worlds beyond. In China, it is used as a symbol in graveyards, and in Native American creation stories it is the turtle that lifts our world into being out of the deep.

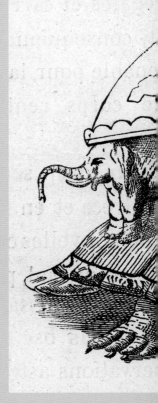

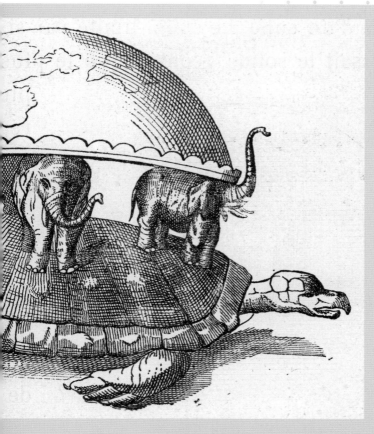

LONGEVITY MIND

Finding your breath

If we're used to the shallow breathing that accompanies a sedentary life, it's harder to connect with the breath. This exercise introduces the basics of deep breathing and shows how to breathe a long and full breath in and out.

1. Lie on your back with knees bent and feet flat on the floor, hip-width apart. Relax your head and shoulders comfortably and rest your hands on your belly, palms down and fingers touching. Rest here until you feel relaxed – you might like a folded blanket beneath your head. Tune in to your breathing. Notice whether your hands move as you breathe.

2. Now inhale as if inflating a balloon in your abdomen from the bottom up. Notice that your abdomen rises and your fingers move apart from each other.

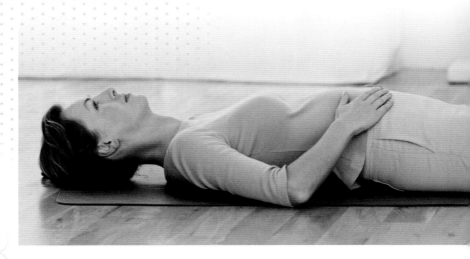

3. Exhale and watch your abdomen sink and your fingers come back to touch. Repeat this full in- and out-breath up to seven times. As you breathe in, notice your ribcage expand to the sides and your back press into the floor. As you breathe out, notice your shoulders descending and a sense of relaxation.

4. Once you feel confident with this lying down, repeat sitting with the back of your pelvis against a wall (you may need to sit on yoga blocks or firm cushions for comfort). Now guide first your shoulder blades and then the back of your head against the wall and look forward. Focus on your breathing and feel your belly and the back of your ribcage swelling with each in-breath.

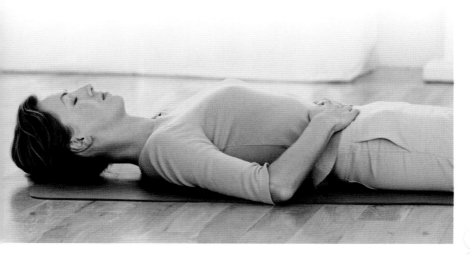

Counting the breath

Your mind may wander during meditation – paying attention is difficult. Counteract this by having a focus to chain your thoughts to and stop them running away from the act of simply sitting. This breath-counting exercise is also useful in preparation for breath-lengthening techniques. The traditional number to aim for is 108!

1. Sit or kneel comfortably upright, hands resting on knees or thighs. Close your eyes. Settle yourself by watching your breath moving in and out for a moment. Feel your ribcage expand with the inhalation and the warmth on your upper lip from the exhalation.

2. When you feel calm, and your breathing has steadied, start counting. Silently say "one" on the first in-breath, and "one" on the first out-breath. Continue counting up, seeing how far

you can get without your attention wandering from the number. Never force the breath. Keep everything really relaxed.

3. When your thoughts wander, return to awareness of your breath, and go back to one. At first you may be able to count to two only, but with perseverance and steady practice you will hit ten or more. Whatever number you reach, notice how you become absorbed and the feeling of calm alertness. This is meditation.

"If the breath is disturbed, the mind is disturbed. By controlling the breath, the yogi gains steadiness of mind. As long as there is breath in the body there is life… therefore we should control the breath."

HATHA YOGA PRADIPIKA,
A 15TH-CENTURY SANSKRIT TEXT ON HATHA YOGA

Lengthening the breath

Learn to breathe like a tortoise! It feels great to stop completely in the pauses between breaths, which brings about a meditative self-awareness.

1. Sit or kneel comfortably upright, hands resting on your knees or thighs. Close your eyes and focus on your breath. Notice it cool as you inhale and warm as you exhale.

2. Inhale for a count of three or four. Then exhale for three or four. This is one cycle. Take a regular breath, if necessary. Repeat three, five or seven cycles.

3. When you feel comfortable with the technique, start to lengthen the out-breath. Inhale for four, then exhale for a count of eight. On the exhalation, let calmness envelop you; then let the in-breath come naturally and easily. If you have to gasp for the in-breath, reduce the length of the hold.

4. Now start to add a pause at the top of the in-breath. Breathe in for four, hold for two, and breathe out for eight. As you pause, retaining the breath, try not to tense or let the shoulders rise, but feel a sense of stillness, clarity and spaciousness. You can increase or decrease the count, but keep to a 2–1–4 pattern.

5. Finally, add another pause, this time at the end of the out-breath. Breathe in for four, hold for two, breathe out for eight and hold for two. Again, if you're gasping for breaths, return to the easier version of the exercise and build up to this final stage slowly.

Three-part breathing

This is another effective way to slow your breathing and allow longer for the exchange of oxygen and carbon dioxide.

1. Sit or kneel comfortably upright, hands resting on your knees or thighs. Close your eyes and watch your breathing until you feel calm and your body has relaxed.

2. Imagine your upper body is a pot, with the base at your pelvis. Inhale for a count of three, filling the bottom third of the pot, around your abdomen. Pause. Continue inhaling for another three counts, filling the centre of the pot, around your chest. Pause. Finally, inhale to the top of the pot, around your shoulder blades, and hold. Let the breath go in one long easy exhalation. This is one cycle. Take a regular breath. Repeat three, five or seven cycles.

3. When you feel ready, which may be in another session, reverse the direction. Take one long easy inhalation, filling your lungs. Exhale for a count of three, emptying the top third of the pot, around your shoulder blades. Pause. Continue exhaling for another three counts, emptying the centre of the pot, around your chest. Pause. Finally, exhale to the very bottom of the pot, around your abdomen, and hold. This is one cycle. Take a regular breath. Repeat three, five or seven cycles.

STOP SMOKING, LIVE LONGER

Smoking is the top preventable cause of morbidity and early mortality – the good news is that it's declining in every age group, and older people seem more able to stay off it. Cognitive ability declines when we breathe polluted air, and smoking pumps that polluted air direct into our age-declining lungs. Giving up smoking makes it easier to breathe, reduces the risk of stroke and cardiovascular disease and stops existing problems becoming more serious. It's a proven way to live longer.

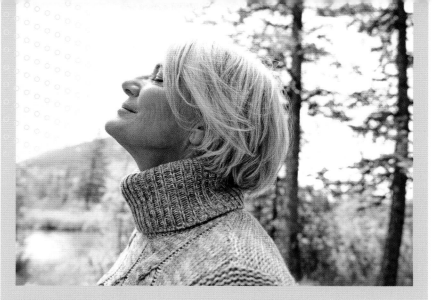

ABOVE: Become aware of the effort you put into the different aspects of breathing, and keep it balanced.

AN EVEN BREATH

In any breathing exercise, notice what happens with each breath from start to finish. Is your breath strong at the start of an inhalation or exhalation but fades toward the end? Try to keep it balanced, so there's as much force at the end of your breath as at the start. You may need to rein it in at the beginning and exert a little more energy at the end to keep the breath smooth and balanced. Work on evening out the length of the in-breath and out-breath by counting the inhalation and exhalation and matching them. You might have to curtail the longer breath.

Notice whether the front of your body expands more than the back. Visualize breathing into the back of your body to even this out. The ribcage extends all around your chest, so should expand evenly. Finally, notice whether your left or right lung feels fuller. Take your awareness to the other lung and see what happens – magically, you can even it out just by thinking about it. That's the power of mindfulness!

A puzzled mind...

...is a sharper mind. Regular mental workouts can help the brain perform as though we're up to ten years younger than our biological age. Like physical exercise, they seem to improve memory and decision-making, quicken reaction times and improve reasoning, verbal-learning and problem-solving skills over the age of 60, when all these can be expected to slow.

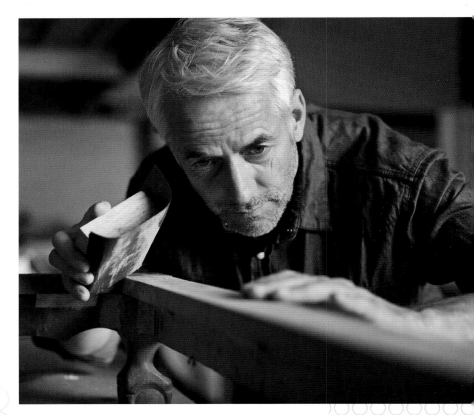

Studies show that people who regularly exercise their brains with stimulating activities, such as crosswords, pastimes that involve learning a skill or an intellectually demanding job, seem less likely to experience cognitive impairment in older age. It's not been proven to prevent dementia, but trials are ongoing. People who engaged with clinical trials also found that brain-training exercises improved their ability to complete everyday tasks, such as shopping.

Improving cognitive function is to do with neuroplasticity – the ability of the brain to change in a sustained way, in structure or function, in response to external stimulation. The ageing brain seems remarkably plastic – look at the many stroke patients who regain function as different parts of the brain take over the roles of damaged areas.

We need to work on preserving our fluid intelligence – core abilities including processing speed, working memory, long-term memory and reasoning. Even if we're educated, which protects us from cognitive ageing, these all decline with age.

How does brain-training work? That's not really known. Some argue that the brain compensates for the losses of ageing by erecting "scaffolding" – additional circuits in the prefrontal area – that helps maintain function. Brain-training helps put up that scaffolding as it encourages us to adapt and reorganize our networks. Others say that by continuing to engage in stimulating study and work, and having a lively lifestyle into older age, we build reserves we can draw on as regular functions decline. New experiences top up our cognitive reservoir.

The key seems to be to keep challenging ourselves rather than settling into a set way of living. Plasticity increases when we push the boundaries and maintain the flexibility to take risks, for example navigating to a new place without using sat nav. Novelty is important – doing something outside our range of life experience is sufficiently challenging to create changes in the brain. Activities that feel tricky and keep pushing us are most beneficial, such as learning a language. While some aspects

LEFT: Mental workouts aren't just for paper or screen; get your body involved, too, in woodworking, crafting or building dry-stone walls.

TIP: Read a book to live longer. In a Yale University study of 3,635 people over 50, those who read for more than 3 hours a week were 23 per cent less likely to die during the 12-year follow-up period than those who didn't read as much. The benefits weren't replicated for reading newspapers.

of language-learning are easier with the experience of age – when we can use life experience and contextual knowledge to make sense of things – others are more demanding. Grammar, mastering idioms that use structures different from our own language, mimicking an accent, which relies on accuracy of hearing, memory and the ability to reproduce – all of these stimulate the executive function, which we need to have in good order so that we can plan, manage time, meet targets and generally organize effectively to get things done. In studies of bilingual students, those who learn a new language in adulthood activate a completely different area of the brain from when using birth languages, showing how cleverly the brain adapts.

Research suggests we need to sustain mental effort over time for durable results. In one study at the University of Regensburg in Germany, people who took up juggling gained volume in the part of the brain that shrinks most in age, the prefrontal cortex, but those who didn't keep it up for three months lost those gains. It looks like we have to do something most days to maintain accrued benefits. Research with video gaming is interesting. The simplest games, such as Tetris, increase response times when played for tens of hours (over watching films). More dynamic action games have even more cognitive-boost power – they quicken our decision-making, hand–eye coordination, visual attention, memory for rules and strategizing because they can be practised happily for hours. And they are – according to research, gamers over 65 play more frequently than any other age group.

PLAY THE MUSIC

A satisfying long-haul way to keep the brain agile is to learn to play an instrument, which requires the coordination of sensory input from eye, ear and hand, and the feedback loop of having to self-correct while performing. The piano is especially effective since it involves both hands working independently while the eye reads and the brain interprets different notation systems for treble and bass clef. In studies, it seems to increase processing speed and hand–eye coordination. The exercising of the hands in themselves is useful, used in stroke rehabilitation. Like learning a language, you can never completely master an instrument, and other long-form problem-solving creative exercises, such as writing a novel, are equally good at providing a stimulating activity we can fall in love with and keep pushing ourselves to get better at – forever. Curiosity, creativity and persistence keep the brain youthful.

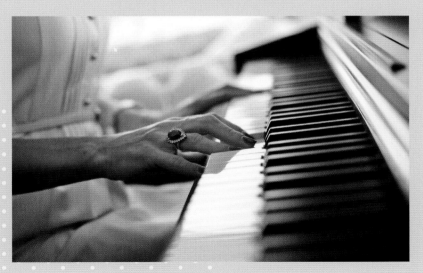

ABOVE: If learning the piano, you'll find it tricky to activate the left hand at first, but dexterity will quickly build.

THE LONDON TAXI DRIVER STUDY

This groundbreaking study showed how amazingly plastic the brain is, even as we age. London taxi-cab drivers (aged 32–62) with many years' experience of navigating the city (including two years learning an encyclopedic number of routes, known as doing "The Knowledge") were compared with a control group of non-taxi drivers. The hippocampus area of the cabbies' brains was completely different from the same area of the non-taxi drivers' brains. In the cabbies it was significantly larger, and those who had been in the job longer had bigger brains in the area connected with spatial awareness. We can significantly increase our grey matter through study and daily practice.

GOOD BRAIN STIMULANTS

- Visit new places and navigate them using a map
- Take up a musical instrument – particularly effective if you don't already play
- Learn a new language
- Try juggling
- Join an orienteering team
- Make up mnemonics – rhymes, acronyms, images or phrases that aid memory
- Join programmes where you read with or mentor young people
- Play memory games
- Cooperate in group problem-solving, such as massive multi-player games
- Immerse yourself in narrative video games with engaging protagonists that build enough empathy and suspense to maintain interest in gameplay over tens of hours
- Knit from a pattern
- Read across a variety of genres and subject areas
- Fiddle away at a daily jigsaw, crossword or sudoku
- Play chess or bridge
- Take a painting class
- Try any craft class that teaches new skills – printmaking, pottery, weaving, spoon carving, upholstery
- Join a creative writing class
- Read or listen to poetry

TIP: Search for online brain-training puzzles, games and apps developed by organizations such as the Alzheimer's Society and GCHQ, or those tested in research studies, such as Game Show, the memory-game app developed by University of Cambridge researchers. Be careful, though – there are many false claims out there, and anyone who claims their product can prevent dementia or Alzheimer's is lying (some companies have been prosecuted).

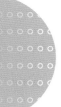

BELOW: Mastering new skills in a form that requires sensitivity, creativity and mindful attention de-stresses while rewiring the brain.

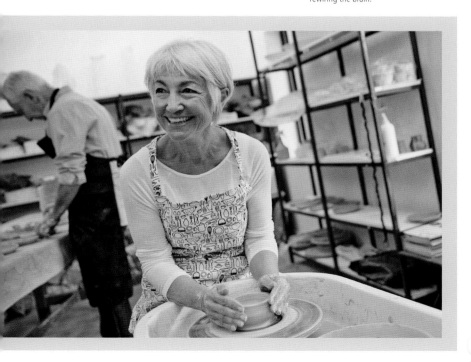

Instant switch-on

Conceived by Moshe Feldenkrais, this is as much a brain challenge as a body-integration exercise. Think of it as a whole-body Rubik's Cube. It challenges you to focus every part of your body and mind on one thing while balancing blocks on your hands and feet as you move. You'll need four paperback books, yoga blocks, beanbags or small feather pillows, plus space to roll around. And a sense of humour!

1. Lie on your back with legs and arms in the air, dead-fly style. Shake them to get rid of tension. Can you roll to your left and over onto your front, holding your hands and feet away from the ground, as if balancing something on them? Try not to put your hands down. You might not get all the way. Once on your front, can you roll back onto your back, keeping your hands and feet raised? Practise a few times, then roll to your right, onto your front, and back again.

2. When you feel ready, balance a book, block or beanbag on one hand and repeat the movement (it's easier with a feather pillow). Try to get onto your front, keeping the object balanced on your hand. Then back again. There's no right way to do it. Try to the left, then the right. Now try with two objects, one on each hand – this can be easier, perhaps because you have to concentrate more fully.

3. Finally, balance objects on one or both feet as well. How far can you get onto your tummy before the books fall? What manoeuvres work to keep you balanced but moving? There is no set solution – let your body instruct you. As you practise, notice how engaged your core muscles are, and how you've switched on attention in every part of the body. You've probably stopped thinking about anything else. After a few days' practice, notice how far you've come with this seemingly impossible task of attention and whole-body engagement. Watch those who've mastered it online – search "full body mobility practice".

> "Man's mind, once stretched by a new idea, never regains its original dimensions."
>
> **OLIVER WENDELL HOLMES**

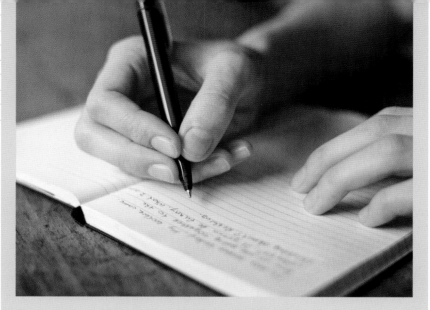

ABOVE: Creative and reflective writing for self-expression has a therapeutic effect.

POETRY PRESCRIPTION

Poetry is the most concentrated form of writing. Each word matters, and the brain-teasing mix of inferred thoughts, the wrestling with imagery and metaphor – when the brain has to jump between literal and surprising meanings – and with intersecting ideas and images, challenges writer and reader to think flexibly and deal with the unexpected. Studies find that listening to poetry stimulates the brain differently from listening to other forms of writing, lighting up areas connected with emotional sensory response while triggering a resting state. The cadences of rhyme and rhythm, the repetition and patterning that bear multiple readings are not only a brain workout, but emotionally rewarding, even healing. In NHS studies, an eight-week course in poetry (or ceramics, drawing or mosaics) resulted in a 37 per cent reduction in GP visits and 27 per cent drop in hospital admissions for those taking part.

The power of questions

Curiosity is one of the markers of longevity, according to many studies – wanting to know how and continuing to ask why, seeking novelty and maintaining an inquisitive interest in other people ensures the brain carries on making new neural pathways.

Curiosity is associated with a healthy central nervous system. It also seems key to maintaining self-esteem and encourages recovery from depression. Continually asking questions means we never stop learning.

Questioning is formalized as a learning technique in the *koan*, an unfathomable question – a riddle with no answer – pondered silently as a form of meditation in the Rinzai Zen tradition. This idea emerged from dialogues between master and student, and was first written down in the 13th century. It is still recommended as a form of brain-training.

When faced with one of these paradoxical statements, the mind goes into overload. There isn't an answer that can be worked out mathematically or using logic, and this creates the beneficial effect. The insoluble nature of such puzzles, the many possibilities and impossibilities it sets in motion, the doubt and frustration, prompt the brain to bypass received knowledge, transcend the apparent paradoxes and jump off on tangents. It deconditions the brain. By just sitting with a *koan* you increase the brain's ability to adapt to new perspectives, be more spontaneous and worry less about getting things right.

"Curiosity is, in great and generous minds, the first passion and the last; and perhaps always predominates in proportion to the strength of the mental faculties."

SAMUEL JOHNSON

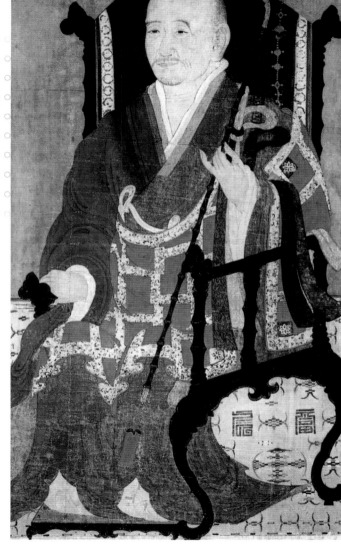

RIGHT: Zen Buddhist practice emphasizes the value of sitting in meditation to free the mind to become conscious of the interconnectedness of everything.

JAPANESE BRAIN-TEASERS

There are no set answers to *koans*, and to try to "solve" them is to lose their essence, which is to stir up and stretch the mind. Don't be tempted to analyse or interpret these examples, just keep calling up the question. Let the problem sit inside you, maturing. You might like to write a poem or make a sketch in response rather than articulating ideas in words.

- Two hands clap and there is a sound. Listen to the sound of one hand clapping.
- Bring me the sound of rain.
- Which direction do you face when you want to move straight ahead?
- What is this?
- What is the treasure in the bag? Keep your mouth closed.

To become, or remain, flexible in mind is an essential factor in increasing neuroplasticity. Tai chi has a concept called double-weightedness – not being wedded to one way of practising but instead being able to adapt, aware of the shift of yin and yang, attentive to where needs to soften and what requires strength to move, and able to shift in new directions on a penny. Any form of movement meditation practice (yoga, dance, capoeira) encourages a widening of awareness, helping us maintain the youthful belief that life offers infinite choices and everything is there for the taking.

Skull-shining breath *(Kapalabhati)*

This yoga cleansing technique, or *kriya*, feels like an internal polishing of the cranium to promote clear-thinking. It is said to encourage perception and wisdom. This technique is thought to support the parasympathetic nervous system while stimulating digestion and brightening the reflexes. Avoid if you have high blood pressure, heart disease or asthma.

1. Settle yourself in a comfortable kneeling or seated position, resting your hands on your thighs or knees. Close your eyes and watch your breath moving in and out.

2. Before starting the breathing technique, place your hands on your lower abdomen, one on top of the other. Take a deep in-breath, then contract your stomach muscles strongly to force the air out of your nose. Notice how the in-breath is naturally sucked into the lungs, like a bellows. This is the technique you'll be using. Try it again. If you're not sure how it works, push your hands into your stomach to encourage the explosive out-breath. If it makes you feel lightheaded, stop the exercise.

3. To start, take a deep breath in, then contract your stomach muscles and puff out the exhalation through your nose. Allow the breath to come in and repeat the rapid out-breath. Repeat the out-breath once a second, allowing the abdomen to relax as the in-breath flows in. There is an in-breath between each puff out. Try not to tense your shoulders and keep your chest relaxed.

4. After five to seven breaths stop – this is one cycle – and return to regular breathing for a minute. Notice how light and bright your skull feels. Repeat two or three rounds, building up to 20 breaths per round.

Horizon-gazing

Try this exercise to widen your perception and gain a sense of spaciousness and appreciation of the possibilities life offers. Alternatively, find a comfortable space outdoors to look up into a wide sky or star-filled night.

1. Sit comfortably upright, hands resting on your knees or thighs. Close your eyes. Focus on the movement of breath in and out. When thoughts or sensations intrude, acknowledge them but ask them to leave. Be patient.

2. Imagine you are sitting on the edge of a cliff, on a hill overlooking a moor or on a wide beach looking out to sea. In your mind's eye watch the horizon; see how wide, distant and open it is. Imagine looking up at the sky, feeling the vast dome arching from horizon to horizon. Sense the spaciousness. You may feel a little dizzy at the scale and expanse.

3. When thoughts occur, visualize them appearing on the horizon, so far away that they no longer have any urgency. Let them slip below the horizon.

4. Take the feeling of expanse and spaciousness within you. Visualize it expanding your internal organs, including your lungs and your brain.

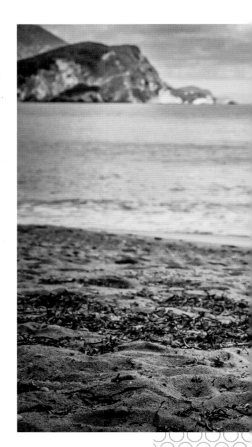

5. Bring yourself back to your body by sensing your sitting bones in contact with the support beneath you. Take your focus to your breath and draw it downward. Feel the inhalation expanding your abdomen and the exhalation drawing your abdomen toward your lower back. Breathe from beneath the ground, imagining the breath seeping up into your feet and sitting bones to earth you. Sit quietly for a few minutes to remove any lasting sensations of dizziness.

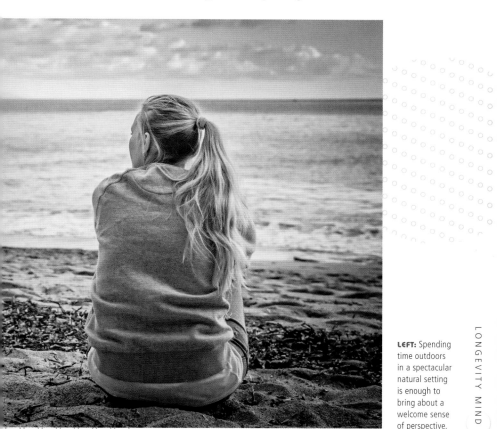

LEFT: Spending time outdoors in a spectacular natural setting is enough to bring about a welcome sense of perspective.

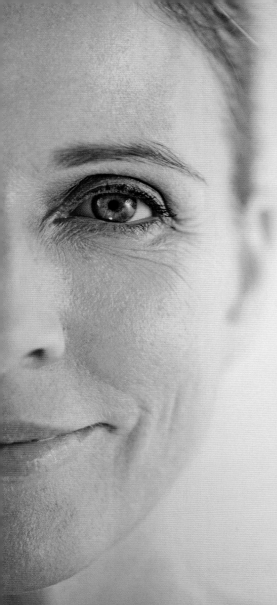

Sensory awareness

As we age, our sensory perception becomes less efficient. Eyesight and hearing fade, our senses of taste and smell lessen, as does the ability to distinguish between scents. We may lose out on touch if we live alone.

LEFT: Yoga teaches that the senses, primarily focused in the face, are distracting. By withdrawing from them we can learn more about who we really are.

This all affects how we relate to other people and our environment, and can rob the brain of stimulus and prevent us from engaging with the kinds of activities that promote longevity. It also leads to increased risk of falls and loss of independence.

Sense-awareness declines because the central nervous system processes stimuli less well in the brain and sense receptors diminish. Scans show that when we are exposed to sensory stimulation, fewer lights are switched on in the relevant areas of the brain as we get older. Sensory dysfunction is also a symptom of neurodegenerative disorders.

The first sense to decline – from as early as our 30s – is our sense of smell. More than three-quarters of people over 80 have an olfactory impairment (half have no sense of smell). That strongly affects our sense of taste – two-thirds of taste sensations are reliant on smell. We also lose taste buds, in number and sensitivity, but at different rates, so while we may taste sweet and bitter, sour becomes less intense and salty declines most.

Even a small loss in our senses of smell and taste can make food seem less appetizing and reduce the amount of saliva we produce, making digestion less efficient. It can contribute to under-nutrition, as does adding extra salt to make food taste better (because we can't taste it as well).

SENSORY TEST

Hold your nose and put a sweet in your mouth. Still holding your nose, suck it for a while and notice what you can taste and which parts of the tongue seem to be stimulated. Now stop holding your nose and breathe in through your nose. Notice how the taste immediately blossoms. That's the affect the olfactory system has on our taste sensations.

TIP: It's worth getting your hearing tested if you find it hard to follow a conversation in a crowded room.

Hearing loss affects older people more than any other chronic condition. As many as 30–50 per cent of us find that it disrupts communication and relationships, leading to frustration and withdrawal into a silent world. This situation may be misdiagnosed as cognitive or behavioural problems. The loss is gradual, so it's difficult to self-diagnose.

Visual acuity tends to be stable until around age 45–50, when it starts to decline. By age 65, half of us need help

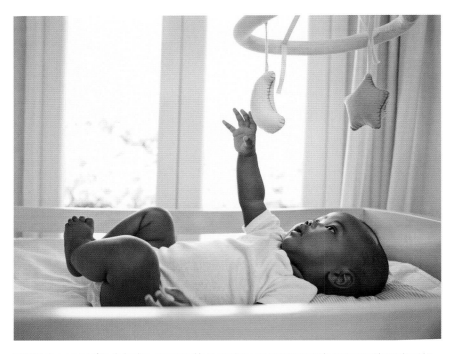

ABOVE: As our sense of touch develops, so we are able to experience our environment and experiment with our place in it.

seeing and find it tricky to focus quickly or adjust to changing light levels. Colours fade and it becomes harder to judge distances and deal with glare. Then there's the effect of conditions such as cataracts, glaucoma and macular degeneration (loss of central vision), all of which are more common after age 65.

Touch is the first sense to develop in the human body and is thought, alongside hearing, to be the final sense to leave us as we die. It extends into the body – the somatosensory system – as well as responding to stimuli from outside. With age, sensitivity declines – along with pain sensation, inside and out – and it takes longer for sensory information about vibration, tactile-sensitivity and temperature to be conducted to the brain. Diabetes can make this worse because it impairs nerve sensitivity. Feet in particular become less sensitive to stimuli and changes in temperature, while older fingers are less able to detect and identify texture. It can take time to react to a touch, but sadly, older people are the least likely to be touched.

So we need as much sensory stimulation as we can get as we age – more light (three times more at 80 than 20) more robust-tasting foods (such as garlic, onions and lemons) and much more touch. Touch is a therapeutic tool all on its own. People who are touched thrive. It lessens anxiety and pain, lowers heart rate and blood pressure, improves the function of the lungs and immunity, increases alertness and brain performance. Above all, it has a positive effect on mood, boosting levels of oxytocin, the "love" hormone. We know that babies who are not touched fail to thrive and may die. And when we engage in thoughtful exercise, we awaken the touch sensors on the inside, too.

BELOW: The body's largest organ, the skin, is exquisitely rich with nerve endings, which when stimulated with therapeutic touch bring about a sense of wellbeing.

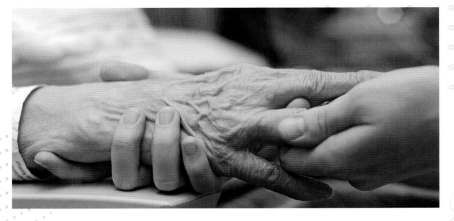

Soothsaying

The Graeae in Greek mythology are a trio of old women, the Old Ones, said to have been born aged with white hair and wrinkled skin. They live in the depths of a cave within a forest at the foot of Mount Atlas, emerging only at night, for darkness is their sensory experience. They have but one eye to share, and pass it between them. And yet they are all-seeing, able to augur the future of young mortals who with their 20/20 vision can see only what's in front of them. Like the third eye (see page 339), the Graeae's is an eye of spiritual perception, giving both inner vision and superhuman clairvoyance.

Many young heroes venture into the forest to look upon their awesome triple-form in search of insight, including Perseus, who steals their eye and wrestles the secret knowledge from the sisters. Now he has their wisdom he seeks out the Gorgons, another three sisters of the Graeae, who live beyond the ocean – the father of both sets of triplets is Phorcys, whom Homer calls "the old man who rules the waves". The Gorgons have eyes so piercing they can turn a man to stone. Perseus severs the head of one of them, Medusa, and the power of her stare is enough to serve as a protective shield. It is mounted on the goddess Athene's breastplate, with replicas set up in public places to ward off evil.

The power of a single eye to see beyond the merely visible and to keep us safe is an emblem used across cultures. It's there as a sign of the all-seeing power and life-giving energy of the sun god Ra, in the Eye of Osiris placed in an embalmed body to guide it through darkness into the light of a new world, and in the Aztec shamans who access the mysteries of the spirit world through the eyes of the jaguar.

RIGHT: An eager Perseus encounters the Graeae. Grey-haired from birth, they share between them one eye and one tooth, yet can see and speak truths from beyond this world.

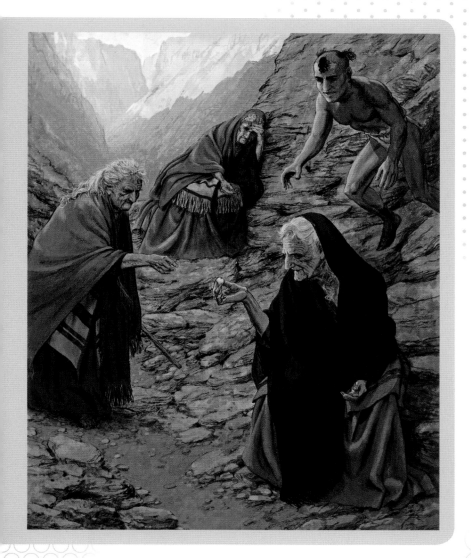

Sense and memory

When we lose our sense of smell – the commonest sense impairment – there are repercussions for memory. Smell is the sense most closely connected to the parts of the brain linked with memory and emotion, the amygdala and hippocampus. Physically, our olfactory "equipment" follows routes close to these areas, and seems to fire the brain more than sight and hearing stimuli do. This limbic system of the brain is very old – it's been with us throughout evolution and is linked with primitive responses. Smell is an emotive and instinctive thing.

Memories triggered by scent seem to stem from our very early years, whereas those prompted by what we see date from later, in early adulthood. Scent memories tend to stay with us into older age, and we have more of them. We seem to remember twice as much with scent impressions as with other memory stimulants. They prompt a sense of travelling back in time, but we can continue to create new memories with scents – by using a new perfume in a new place, for example.

Many forms of meditation work by switching on the senses. If we can awaken our senses of sight, sound and scent, and dwell on tempting touch and taste, we will be brought instantly in contact with what's happening here and now, and can appreciate the immediacy and diversity of the world in this way stimulates the brain.

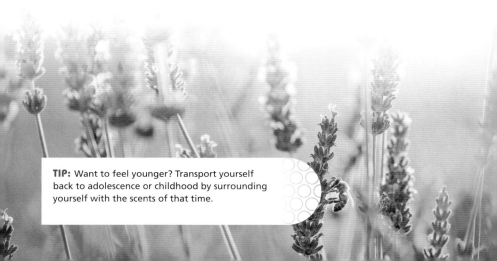

TIP: Want to feel younger? Transport yourself back to adolescence or childhood by surrounding yourself with the scents of that time.

Sight meditation

Mindful attention to what's going on in front of the eyes expands our awareness and can feel like having new young vision. Find a special quiet place to sit and watch the world, or combine this exercise with Mindful Walking (see page 280).

1. Sit or kneel in a comfortable upright position outdoors, hands resting on knees or thighs. Centre your head on top of your spine and keep your eyes alert. Close your eyes and calm yourself by watching breath flow in and out of your nostrils.

2. Open your eyes and look at the scene in front of you as if for the first time. Note the real colours rather than the storybook hues we imagine the world to have – the sky isn't blue, grass is more than green, a concrete wall is a rainbow of tones. Understand the sights as visual impressions without labels, like an Impressionist painting.

3. Bend forward and examine a blade of grass or stone in close-up. Then look to the horizon and try to decipher the specks. Point your chin to the sky and let its vastness widen your perspective. Without moving your shoulders, turn your head to look behind you, with every out-breath increasing the rotation.

4. Imagine seeing the scene through the eyes of a dog or an alien. Then blur your senses by trying to imagine the sensations a flower would perceive from here. Let your eyesight free your mind from the impoverished nature of regular perception.

Incense meditation

You can do this exercise with favourite perfumes or the contents of a spice box, but incense is used across cultures as an aid to meditation. You will need some incense and a notebook.

1. Light some incense and place it in front of you, perhaps on a low table. Sit or kneel comfortably with spine erect, resting your hands on your knees or thighs. Close your eyes. Take your gaze inside and watch your breath moving in and out. Feel the warm exhalation on the top of your upper lip and let each in-breath come naturally.

2. When you feel calm and grounded, start to notice the scent of the incense. Let everything else drift away. When thoughts intrude, accept them without reacting and return again and again to the scent. Can you discern the top and base notes? How does the initial effect differ from the lasting impression? Taste the scent on your palate.

3. Listen to what the scent has to say, however hard this might be. How do you respond to it emotionally? Does it remind you of a time, place or person?

4. Now try to write a description of each scent. A list is fine. Try to avoid clichés; can you find new ways of describing the elements of the scent? Is it useful to think of them as sounds or colours?

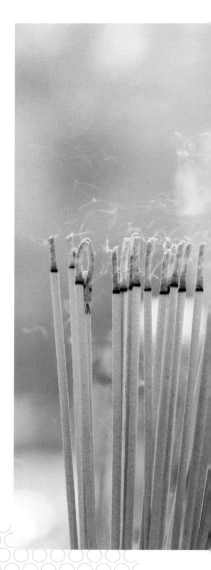

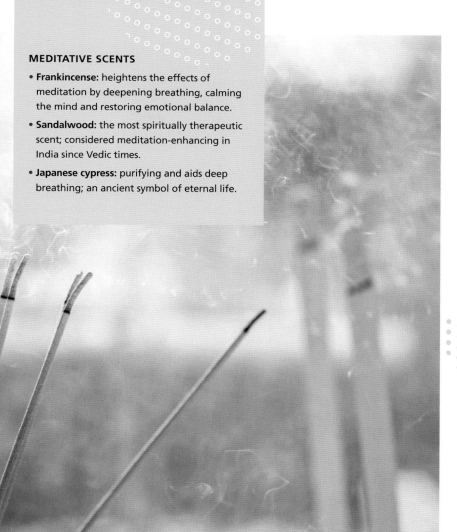

MEDITATIVE SCENTS

- **Frankincense:** heightens the effects of meditation by deepening breathing, calming the mind and restoring emotional balance.

- **Sandalwood:** the most spiritually therapeutic scent; considered meditation-enhancing in India since Vedic times.

- **Japanese cypress:** purifying and aids deep breathing; an ancient symbol of eternal life.

Body memories

Memories are held in body as well as mind. This exercise helps recall the sensation of past experiences, and can be surprisingly intense. It allows you to experience a sense of touch from within. You might like to write down thoughts that occur after practising this exercise.

1. Lie on your back with feet on the floor, hip-width apart. Relax your arms away from your sides, palms up. Relax your back, shoulders and back of the head into the support beneath you. Extend your legs, if that feels comfortable, and let your feet flop outward.

2. Think about a time when you felt rapture. That's the emotion that takes us outside ourselves. It's a feeling of awe and wonder in something bigger, whether in nature (sunrise, mountain peaks), a religious experience (a cathedral, mass) or human acts of creation (a piece of music, great work of art). Take yourself back to that moment; notice how your body responds, which parts are activated. You may sense butterflies in your stomach or a sense of dropping down. Bathe in the sensations for as long as feels comfortable. Then let those feelings go.

3. Think about a time when you felt pleasure. Pleasure is focused on ourselves. It's the feeling that comes with a favourite food or drink, sinking into a warm bath or the sensation of silk on skin, or an oiled hand sweeping over your back. Now take yourself back to that moment; notice how your body responds. Maybe there's a feeling of warmth and connection. Which parts of your body are affected? Enjoy the internal sensations for as long as feels good. Let those feelings settle in your body. Then let them go.

4. Come back to an awareness of the breath. Feel the back of your head, your shoulders, your pelvis, your heels on the floor. Roll to one side and rest. Take your time to come to, before pushing yourself up to sitting.

RIGHT: The Cathedral Basilica of the Assumption in Covington, Kentucky, USA. The atmosphere of a holy place can make a sense of rapture seem tangible.

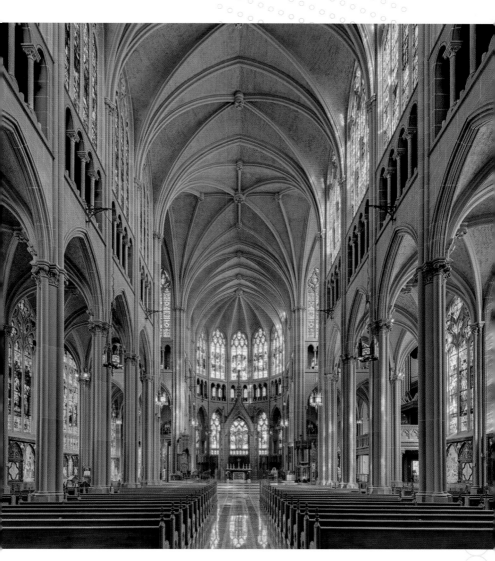

Sound meditation

Sharpen your hearing by tuning in to surrounding sounds that we usually zone out.

1. Wherever you are, stop what you're doing, stand or sit up straight and shut down all your senses but your hearing. It helps to close your eyes.

2. Focus on the sounds immediately surrounding you. What can you hear with your left ear? What sounds can you catch with your right ear? What can you hear in front of you? Now behind you? Don't focus on pleasant sounds; note the blaring siren, a car alarm, a shout, a whining child. Don't label the sounds, just differentiate them by tone and timbre.

3. Now listen outside your immediate surroundings. What can you hear beyond you; what sounds are in the building? What can you hear outdoors? Try to extend your hearing beyond the traffic and the birdsong, the wind and the rustling of trees. In meditation we are encouraged to tune in to the inaudible and sense the universe humming.

BELOW: Listen for birdsong – it can be audible in the most unlikely of settings. Which songbirds can you recognize?

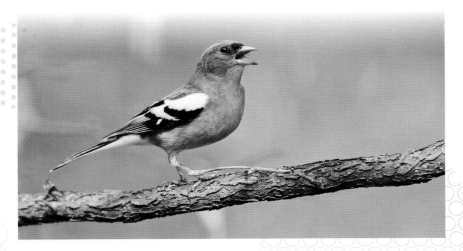

Colour breathing

Choose a colour – deep blue for calming, turquoise for energizing, silver for healing. As you breathe in through your nose, visualize the colour flowing in down the back of your throat. As you exhale, imagine it running across the back of your shoulders (feel them broaden) and down your arms into your soft extended fingers and out into the universe.

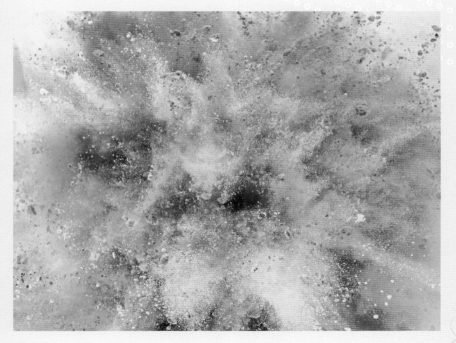

Barefoot walking

The feet contain a wealth of nerve-endings, and pressure sensors connect them with every part of the body. We can use them to awaken the senses in this moving meditation based on the Japanese tradition of takefumi – walking on bamboo – as used by Samurai warriors, who equated the sole with the soul. It challenges the feet with unexpected combinations of textures. You will need to set aside some space outdoors.

1. Prepare a walking meditation pathway by assembling trays of different textured objects in a row – maybe gravel, varying-sized pebbles, grass, sand, mud, very warm water, icy water, lengths of bamboo cut in half, rounded side up, broom handles.

2. Stand at the start of the path and centre yourself by standing upright, bodyweight balanced between both feet, spine straight and crown of the head pulling toward the sky. Watch your breath moving in and out.

3. Start walking along the path. Carefully ease your bodyweight onto each new surface, paying attention to sensations and watching how different parts of the foot react. Experiment by shifting your bodyweight, rocking from side to side and forward and back.

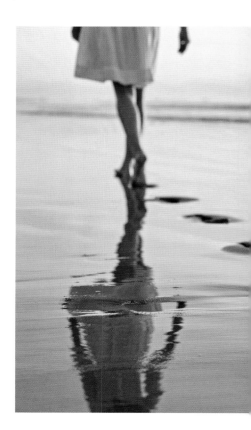

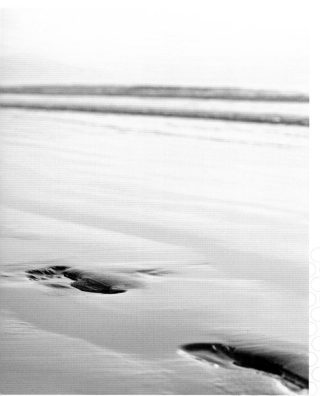

4. When you tire of one sensation, move to the next station. Notice how the rest of your body responds to the changing stimuli. When thoughts intrude, breathe them away and return to the sensations in your feet. Practise for five to ten minutes once a week.

Power of tango

Numerous studies attest to the power of dance as an aid to longevity, not only in making the body physically stronger and better coordinated, but in keeping brain and social needs stimulated. It's the only physical activity associated with a lowered risk of dementia, and dancing tango seems to have benefits all its own – practitioners report dropping into a state of flow, total mindful awareness that blocks out everything else, including the passage of time. Research suggests that tango might help balance and memory-loss more than comparable forms of exercise. So well recognized are its beneficial effects for people with Parkinson's (more than standard physiotherapy) that free classes are offered to patients in Buenos Aires.

The improvisational element is important – this is not a choreographed form. Instead, we respond to the touch of a partner, pick up on emotional clues, interpret signals in the music and lyrics, mark the bodies of other couples and send millisecond decisions from brain to body that rewire our neural circuits, preserving cognitive function.

Then there's the spiritual aspect – dancers talk of a spirit speaking or dancing through them, of a trance-like connection with the mysterious roots of tango and its relationship with the African god Chango, ancestor of virility and strength. The tango is a heart-focused form. First you learn to walk with your hand touching your partner's heart; that demands a sincere connection and mutual respect, the sensitivity to understand and respond to another person without using words. It's this that is danced – not learned steps.

The heart leads the connection with the music, too. It's a yearning form suited to older age that speaks of memories, the sadness of time gone and opportunities lost. It can be an erotic expression (certainly tango has been shown to raise levels of testosterone in men and women) and the passion in motion is accessible regardless of age or physical condition. This brings confidence – a dance of honour and prestige empowers its dancers and self-assurance comes when we are in command of a repertoire of movements and the gift of grace.

RIGHT: In tango we establish a connection heart-to-heart before learning the steps. It's about the power of reading a partner and communicating without words.

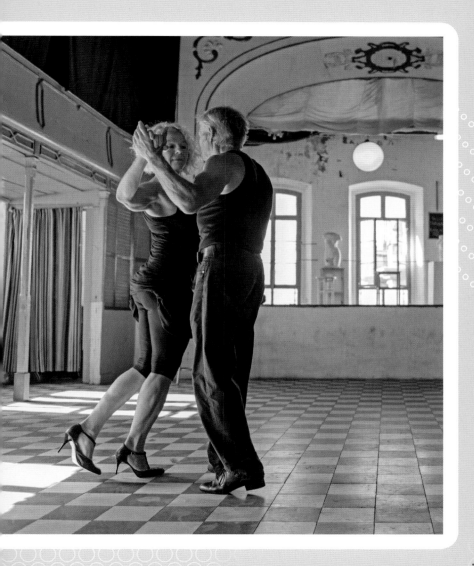

Part 4

LONGEVITY SPIRIT:
energy, faith, connection

The word "spirit" derives from the Latin *spiritus*, meaning breath and soul; it is the principle that animates us and imparts our essential nature. Spirit is our vitality and energy force, but also carries the sense of an inspiring power greater than us, the essence of a place or community, and what's left after the fading of the corporeal being.

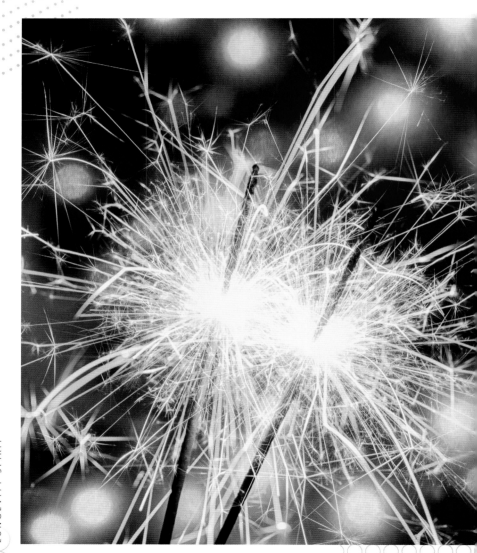

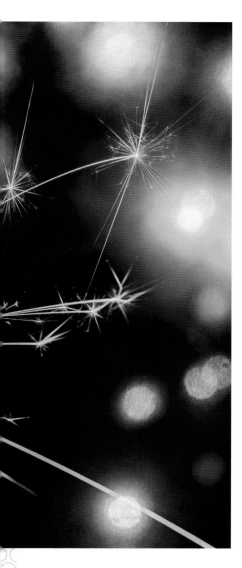

What is the spirit of good ageing? It's the maintaining of our character and vitality – what makes us "us" – as the decades pass, and refining how we relate to this core nature as we face change and loss.

Energy can occupy us more as we age. Loss of energy is a major symptom of midlife, associated with menopause and its male version, andropause (a decline in testosterone production affects 20 per cent of men over 60). A declining metabolism may be to blame – the process that combines fuel from what we eat with oxygen to produce the energy that powers us.

Happily, for many women life post-menopause is injected with new zest and lust for living (and maybe also actual lust). Anthropologist Margaret Mead named this surge of physical and psychological energy "postmenopausal zest" (PMZ) back in the 1950s, while one of the 20th century's most inspirational yoga teachers, Vanda Scaravelli – who only started teaching yoga in her 60s – compared this "re-awakening" to flowers that bloom in the autumn. It seems to arrive with the settling of hormones after the rocky ride of menopause and stabilizing levels

LEFT: The spark of life burns brightly if you keep it well fed with joyful activities and by connecting with people who make you feel good.

of testosterone. It's probably the first time since primary school that women are free of fluctuating hormones – the energy, confidence and assertiveness of the ten-year-old tomboy can be incredibly empowering, sparking the drive to start businesses, run marathons, stand for public office. Research shows rates of depression in women decrease post-menopause: an NHS study found we're more likely to be depressed in our 20s than in our 50s, while a longitudinal study from Melbourne University found that negative mood and depression in women reduced significantly as women moved from mid- to later life. British Psychological Survey data suggests that women feel more content at 60 than at 40, and in a Danish study into women's positive experiences of menopause, participants mentioned the opportunities it brought for personal growth and the freedom to pursue what made them feel good. This new-found energy and serenity might coincide with children leaving home, a rethinking of life's purpose, and freedom from the stressful body stereotypes of our reproductive years. Office for National Statistics data show people in the UK are happiest between the ages of 65 and 79.

For many people, spirit is about awareness of the divine and connecting with energy outside ourselves. Research finds clear health benefits for older people who express a faith, and spirituality seems to support the journey into very old age, with its loss of self-sufficiency and agency.

Most of all, spirit is about finding contentment in how and where we live and with whom we spend our lives. In places around the world where longevity seems to be a cultural habit – the islands of Okinawa, the Seventh Day Adventist community in Loma Linda, California, for instance – over and again we see a community that shares values and a way of life that's close, spiritually nourishing and supports everyone. This, in the end, can empower us to let go in serenity, in the knowledge that life has been good and we have passed on what we can so that future generations can also lead a good life – our energetic legacy.

TIP: Visit a doctor if lack of energy, insomnia or loss of appetite is a problem – these can be signs of depression, often missed in older people.

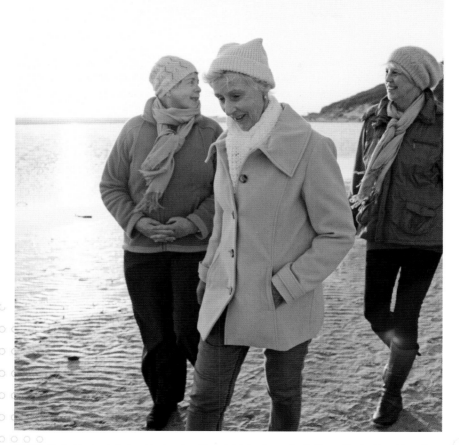

ABOVE: Having friends – both close friends and a wider social circle – is associated with cognitive health and longevity.

What is energy?

Conventional medicine, Ayurveda and Traditional Chinese Medicine have different notions about the nature of energy, how it changes as we age, and ways to rebalance and make the most of what we have.

In Western medicine, energy expenditure is tied up with our metabolic rate, which declines with age as our body mass reduces and tissue function decreases. Researchers are working to understand the role of metabolism in longevity. In 1908, German scientist Max Rubner posited a neat theory. He observed that small mammals with a higher metabolism wear out their life span more quickly than larger ones that use less energy per body mass. He suggested that each species is allocated a specific amount of energy, and how quickly it's used up determines length of life. It's called the "rate of living" theory. Unfortunately, it's not that simple. Larger species with a slower metabolism do seem to live longer than higher-metabolism small species – but we don't know why and can't extrapolate to individual lives.

What we do know is that activity (even fidgeting), good sleep and a healthy diet keep the metabolism active. Our resting metabolic rate – responsible for up to 80 per cent of our energy expenditure – slowly falls after the age of 20, perhaps connected with a loss of mass in our organs, brain, muscles and bone as we

age. Exercise is protective because it keeps us building muscle and bone. In studies, older women in particular who trained long-term as runners or swimmers didn't see a decline in their resting metabolic rate; it matched that of young competitive runners. Going back to the rate of living theory, in human studies, neither energy expenditure nor resting metabolism seemed to predict life span, but those in the lowest third of activity levels were three times more likely to die than those in the top third. It seems that being more active preserves energy and life span.

In the Indian and Chinese traditions, the life force or subtle energy that enlivens us – all life forms are thought to be a manifestation of this universal spirit – is known as *prana* or *qi*. Both encompass the meanings "breath" and "energy". This life force circulates in the universe, but also in our bodies where its presence powers our breathing, circulation and cellular processes. It flows through subtle channels known as *nadis* in the Indian tradition and *meridians* in the Chinese. At the major intersections of these channels we find powerful chakra energy centres in the Indian system (*dantiens* in the

Chinese). The main ones are sited along a central energy channel running parallel with the spine. Blockage in one energy channel means energy is stuck, causing depletion elsewhere. By practising yoga and tai chi or qigong, meditation and breath-awareness, we become aware of the subtle energy circulating. These practices diffuse blockages and allow energy to flow freely, bringing balance, vigour and strength to the whole system and promoting healing and long life.

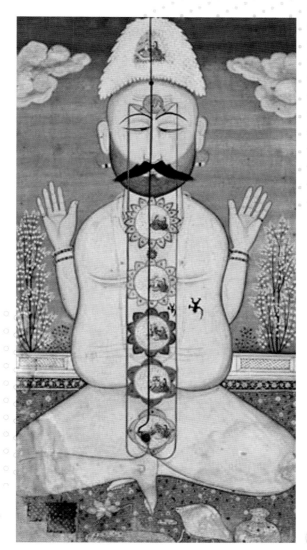

RIGHT: The chakra energy centres running up from the base of the spine to the crown of the head, depicted in an 18th-century illustration.

AYURVEDIC ENERGY-BALANCING

Ayurveda sees the body as a mix of three *doshas*, or constitutional energies – *vata*, *pitta* and *kapha* (see page 17). We are said to have more *vata* energy in the later decades. Excess *vata* is associated with many conditions associated with ageing, such as fatigue, insomnia, digestive problems, dry skin, cold hands and feet. *Vata* energy is exacerbated by lack of a routine or nourishing food, and eased by qualities of *pitta* (warmth) and *kapha* (oiliness and stillness). To reduce *vata*:

- Establish a set routine.
- Massage the body with sesame oil.
- Stimulate the scalp with coconut oil.
- Wrap up warm.
- Slow down and rest.
- Eat more sweet, sour and salty tastes (see page 258).
- Eat enough dairy, nuts and rice
- Cook with warming spices, such as ginger and garlic, cinnamon and turmeric.
- Practise Inverted Pose (*Viparita Karani*, see page 342).
- Rebalance with Alternate Nostril Breath (*Nadi Shodhana Pranayama*) (see page 344).

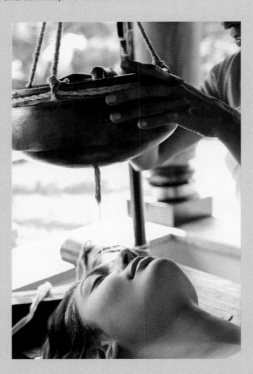

ABOVE: In a Shirodhara Ayurvedic treatment, a stream of warm, herb-infused oil is poured onto the chakra centre at the third eye.

Feel the energy

By performing movements with mindfulness, we can become aware of *qi* – in this qigong exercise, feel it between the palms. You might sense *qi* energy (referred to as *prana* in the yoga tradition, or the energy of life) as a tingling in the hands, or feel that the space between your palms is somehow thicker than usual. If you don't feel anything, keep trying; it can take practice to tune in your awareness.

1. Stand in the basic qigong pose, feet a little more than hip-width apart and knees soft. Relax your shoulders and release tension in your neck and face.

2. Bring your palms together in front of you, and rub briskly for 30 seconds. Shake your hands, then repeat the rubbing for another 30 seconds. Now release your palms and imagine a small ball between them. Can you feel it? Move your hands out slightly and in again, to see if you can sense it. This is your electromagnetic field.

3. Inhaling, slowly pull your palms apart – can you feel the ball of energy growing? Stop when you can no longer feel the energy field.

4. Exhaling, push your palms toward each other as if squeezing the ball of energy. Can you feel it becoming more intense? The more you slow down and focus on the movement, the more likely you are to feel the sensation of *qi*. Repeat the slow pulling and pushing seven times or more.

Nectar of immortality

Does yoga help us access an energetic font of immortality? Many long-lived teachers attest to its powers of preserving body and mind. The 20th century's leading teachers achieved great ages, teaching until the end: BKS Iyengar lived to 95, K Pattabhi Jois to 93, Vanda Scaravelli to 91, Indra Devi to 102 and their own teacher, Krishnamacharya, to 100.

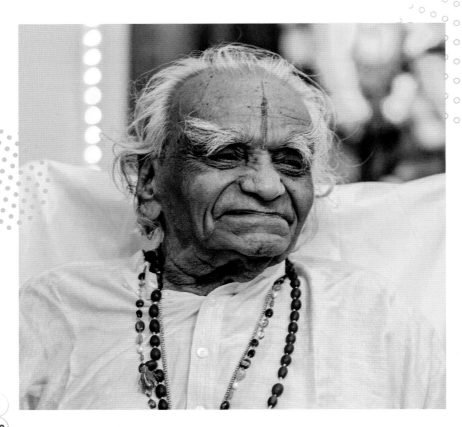

The *Hatha Yoga Pradipika*, a 15th-century Sanskrit text on Hatha Yoga, tells of a divine "nectar of immortality", *amrita*, that arises near the *soma* chakra, a subtle-energy point on the top and toward the back of the head – where you'd wear a high ponytail or man-bun – above the soft palate. This is said to be the elixir of life, ensuring perfect health and extending life. We cultivate it through meditation and yoga postures. Over decades, the daily grind causes this rejuvenating fluid slowly to drip away, down the channel between nose and throat and on down through the chakra energy centres to *manipura* chakra around the solar plexus, where it is consumed by *agni*, digestive fire.

The position of the soma chakra corresponds to the site of the pineal gland (17th-century philosopher Descartes called it the seat of the soul) which synthesizes serotonin and melatonin. Most active in darkness, it controls our circadian rhythms and sleep-wake cycle. In some species it resembles an eye, and has been referred to as a third eye because of its ability to respond to, and transduce, light.

Specific yogic techniques are designed to stop this nectar of immortality ebbing away. Inverted postures conserve the vital fluid in the upper body; chin "locks" (when the chin is lowered after exhaling fully to "seal in" subtle energy or *prana*) capture the essence in the throat and direct energy back upward. Any techniques that cultivate stillness and a peaceful heart allow us to tap into this well of potential and develop vitality and vigour. Many techniques focus on the throat, the site of *vishuddha* chakra, which is connected with communication, our power to choose our life course, speak up for ourselves, and develop a spiritual voice. In terms of conventional medicine, this area corresponds with the thyroid and parathyroid glands, which secrete hormones governing the functioning of every system and cell in the body, influencing everything from muscle strength to memory and metabolism.

LEFT: BKS Iyengar, one of the 20th century's most important yoga teachers, talked of old age revealing the stability (*sthira*) and sweetness (*sukham*) of body, intelligence and self as he practised and held the postures.

"The yogi who drinks the soma juice with a concentrated mind, doubtlessly conquers death"

HATHA YOGA PRADIPIKA

Preserving vital energy

This is quite an advanced breathing technique, so if you feel breathless at any point, return to regular deep breathing. Practise first without holding your breath or gazing inward.

1. Sit comfortably on your heels (or on a chair) and rest your palms on your thighs or knees. Take a deep breath in, feeling your abdomen expand.

2. Open your mouth and stick out your tongue, down toward your chin. Exhale fully, making a long "haaaa" sound.

3. At the end of the out-breath, curl up your tongue and rest the tip at the top of your palate. Close your mouth and tuck in your chin slightly. Hold the out-breath, gazing between your eyebrows if you can.

4. Relax your gaze, lift your chin, release your tongue and allow the in-breath to come in naturally through your nose. Take a regular breath. Repeat twice if comfortable.

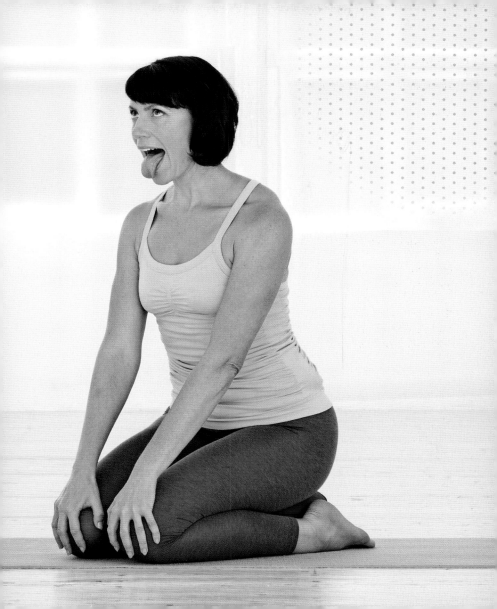

Inverted pose *(Viparita Karani)*

This restorative yoga inversion conserves energy and is said in the ancient yoga texts to promote longevity by stimulating *amrita*, "youth dew". If you feel the cold, wear warm socks and cover yourself in a blanket. The pose is reassuring if you feel dragging in the pelvic organs and is said to be helpful for hair loss. You will need a firm bolster or two yoga blocks.

1. Sit sideways to a wall, with one shoulder and one knee beside the wall. Carefully swivel around, leaning backward and supporting yourself behind with your hands as you guide your buttocks toward the wall and swing your legs up the wall.

2. Lie back, resting your back and shoulders on the floor. The back of your pelvis should feel well supported on the floor. If this is not comfortable, or if you like the support, lift your hips and place a yoga block or firm bolster under your pelvis. Lie back so that your tailbone rests in the gap between your support and the wall. Check that your head, chest and legs are aligned, and not leaning to one side or the other. If uncomfortable, shuffle back to give yourself more space. Relax your arms by your sides, palms up, or rest them on the floor behind you. Close your eyes and relax for at least 8 and up to 15 minutes.

3. To exit the pose, bend your knees and place the soles of your feet on the wall. Push into your feet to lift your buttocks, and slide the bolster or blocks to the side. Return your buttocks to the floor and roll sideways. Rest on your side, before pushing gently with your hands into a sitting position.

4. For total relaxation, strap your thighs with a yoga belt. Keeping your legs in position reduces the amount of effort you put in and can feel very calming. Cover the eyes with an eye pillow to release tension in the face, and place eye pillows or small sandbags on the palms. The pressure feels very comforting.

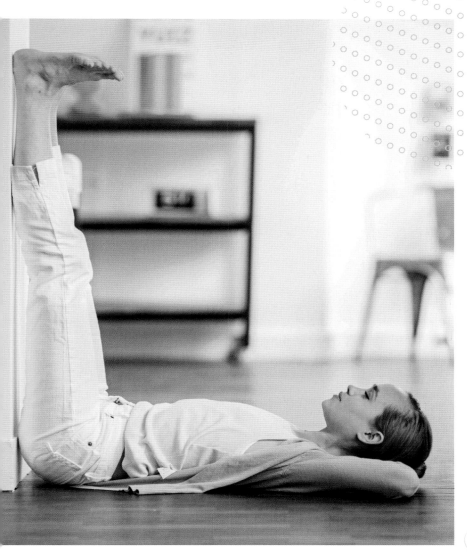

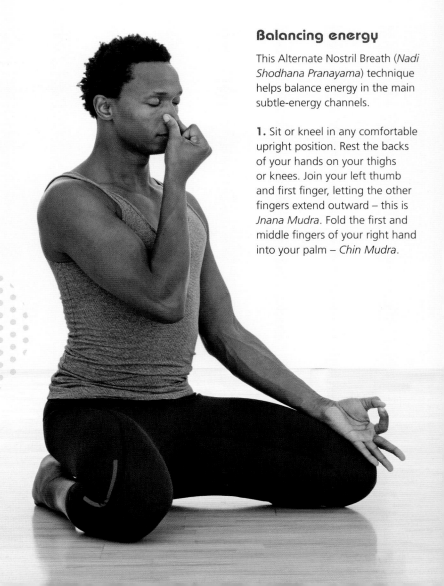

Balancing energy

This Alternate Nostril Breath (*Nadi Shodhana Pranayama*) technique helps balance energy in the main subtle-energy channels.

1. Sit or kneel in any comfortable upright position. Rest the backs of your hands on your thighs or knees. Join your left thumb and first finger, letting the other fingers extend outward – this is *Jnana Mudra*. Fold the first and middle fingers of your right hand into your palm – *Chin Mudra*.

2. Take your right hand to your nose. Place the ring and little fingers on your left nostril, thumb on your right nostril.

3. Close your eyes. Inhale through both of your nostrils, then block your left nostril with the ring and little fingers and exhale through your right nostril. Inhale through your right nostril, envisaging activating energy.

4. At the top of the inhalation, block your right nostril with the thumb and exhale through your left nostril. Inhale through your left nostril, feeling a cooling calming energy. This is one cycle. Repeat up to seven cycles. Finish on an exhalation from the right nostril, then inhale through both nostrils.

TIP: Try cooling lunar breathing, inhaling through your left nostril and exhaling through the right each time, thought to stimulate the "cave" from which *amrita* seeps. For warming solar breathing, inhale through your right nostril and exhale through the left. This is thought to counter excess *vata* as we age by stimulating *pitta* and *kapha* energy.

The power of faith

Belief seems to help us live longer, healthier lives. Research suggests that people with spiritual beliefs are better at coping with stress and chronic illness, experience less pain and recover from illness more quickly than those with no beliefs.

The act of regularly attending religious services may add seven years to life, one study found, and the beneficial effects of faith seem particularly marked in women.

Most research has been carried out in traditional religious communities with a specific system of beliefs, ideals for living and formal ways of coming together, much of it in Christian communities in the US with easily observable patterns of worship. In the UK, there has been a marked decline in numbers professing a traditional religious affiliation. Church-goers are considerably older than the wider public, peaking between 65 and 74, and there has been a significant increase in the proportion of people over 50 or 60 applying for the ministry.

It may be the more formal aspect of worship and its social connections that produce the beneficial effects. The word "religion" derives from the Latin *religare*, "to tie or bind". We are bound as one by shared beliefs with those in our community now, those who went before and those yet to come. We might join a congregation for personal reasons, but soon find that worship comes with a ready-made web of relationships, roles and duties we can slot into.

The world's religions teach that we cannot thrive on our own, that we are part of something greater – if we trust without reservation that we are all made in the image of God, then we are held at the centre of a relationship with the divine and every other created being. As we age and we begin to face challenges in being self-sufficient, this can feel more relevant. Studies of older people in care homes found their image of God was important in bringing meaning to life and they had reflected on it more than people living independently. Researchers suggest this might result from increased feelings of frailty, spending longer "being" rather than "doing", depending on others for agency and having more time alone to look within and reflect on life so far. A connection with God seemed to take the place of relationships with people, after a move to a care home and increasing isolation from friends and family.

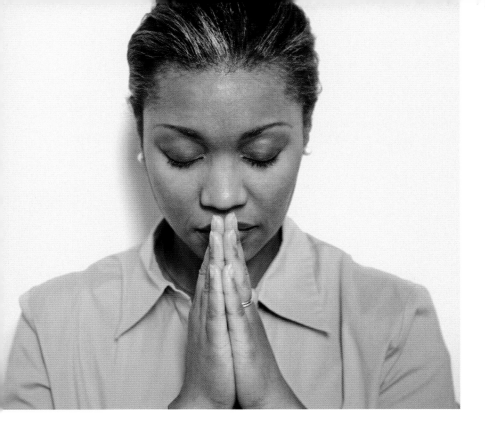

Spiritual awareness in general can help us come to terms with the facts of ageing – we will become physically frailer, our brain power will dwindle and we will come to depend on others. It helps us see ageing as a journey, that we don't develop a "set" self in, say, early adulthood. We have the capacity to develop throughout life, to keep finding new purpose and understanding of what it is to be alive.

ABOVE: When we bring our hands together and close our eyes, whether in formal prayer or simple contemplation, we acknowledge our human need for a sense of meaning.

Studies confirm that we become more spiritual as we age, even if we opt out of a formal religious framework – meditation, mindfulness and awareness-movement practices encourage us to find a place of inner silence in the present that brings insight into who we are in essence, when physical capacity and memory are stripped away.

A spiritual life can provide meaning and hope in the face of increasing absence (of ability, agency, people, places). It allows us to transcend the personal self and appreciate the interconnectedness of all things. It offers compassionate ways to come to terms with the effects of the passing of time and the coming

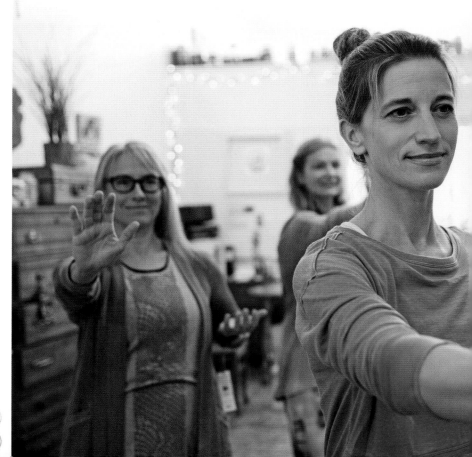

of the end, including the possibility of reconciliation. It has an important role in "dignity therapy" in end-of-life care. A spiritual life allows us space to articulate who we are becoming and eases the frustration or regret that can bring.

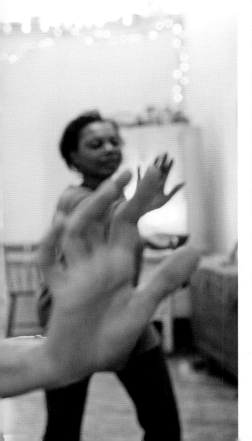

THE TREASURE OF *SHEN*

In Traditional Chinese Medicine, *shen*, or spiritual energy, is the least tangible of the three essential forces of life – with *qi* and *jing* (see page 18), *shen* forms the three treasures we must keep in balance to ensure health and longevity. Stored in the upper *dantien*, around the third eye (see page 339), *shen* is said to be evident as a sparkle in the eye. Stores are depleted through the eyes, too, and when this energy is out of balance, it manifests in anxiety and mental instability. We nourish and add to our reservoir of *shen* through meditation and introspection, as well as by practising qigong.

LEFT: A mindful physical practice, such as qigong or yoga, can offer an awareness of the spiritual dimension and the support of a congregation of like-minded souls.

Advent of longevity

Another "Blue Zone" community – one of five highlighted as a world centre of longevity – is based in the town of Loma Linda, California. People here live four to ten times longer than the average Californian, and have the longest average life expectancy in the US (88 for men, 89 for women).

Longevity may be connected with the close-knit nature of the community – the people we spend most time with determine whether we age well by affirming our good (or bad) lifestyle choices. Many of the world's longest-lived communities are isolated in some way – on islands and peninsulas, caught between mountain and ocean, hemmed in by ethnic barriers and warring neighbours. Here it's by religious practice – one third of the community are Seventh Day Adventists. Life is lived in accordance with strict principles (which happen to be very healthy) – food is vegetarian and unprocessed, including plenty of nuts, and people enjoy community meals. Exercise is valued and built into neighbourhoods, rest and de-stressing encouraged (the Sabbath is fiercely observed). Smoking is discouraged. So while spirituality plays a role in longevity, it's the practical aspects of community life that really make a difference – especially the will of the community to do the right thing to make this place and the wider world better for everyone.

Psychiatrist Harold G Koenig researches the effects of religion and spirituality on health. In work with older people he found that when certain spiritual needs were met, healthy ageing was more likely. Perhaps unsurprisingly, these spiritual needs included religious needs, such as the need to experience a relationship with a living God, to express ourselves in a religious way and to have our religious world-view respected. However, these needs also encompassed wider spiritual requirements, such as to be supported when we face loss, to forgive and be forgiven, to have space to express anger and doubt, to serve others and feel gratitude, to transcend

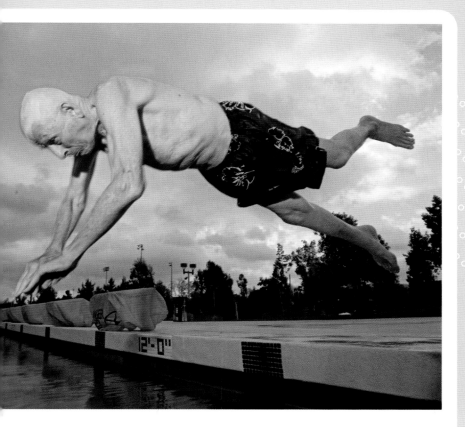

our circumstances and to prepare well for death. Underpinning everything, therefore, are the basic human needs for unconditional love, for dignity and self-esteem, and for a meaningful life that contains hope.

ABOVE: A 94-year-old man takes his daily swim in Loma Linda, California, a town renowned for the great age and good health of its inhabitants.

Breathing the universe

The effect of this centuries-old yoga breathing technique is to transcend the personal and experience the interconnection of all things and the world of spirit. With each in-breath repeat the sound "*So*", on the out-breath repeat "*Hum*". It's that simple. Start whispering the words to get used to their sound, then repeat them silently. "*So*" signifies oneself and is said to be the sound made by every living creature when inhaling; "*Hum*" refers to the universe, and is the sound all creatures make when exhaling. By repeating the two words over and over with the inhalation and exhalation of *prana*, breath and life energy, you link yourself with the energy of the world and every living thing in it.

RIGHT: By contemplating the universe we align ourselves with natural forces, the cycle of life and the cosmic energy of circadian rhythms.

Compassion meditation

There's evidence that we have an increased facility to be prayerful and reflective as we age. Compassion is a quality that evolves, and older people are the spiritual engine of many faith communities, playing the role of spiritual parent or prayer companion. This practice, *Metta Bhavana*, develops our innate compassion, kindness, tolerance and empathy as we cultivate loving kindness for all beings. Break it down into ten-minute sessions, becoming comfortable with each step before moving to the next.

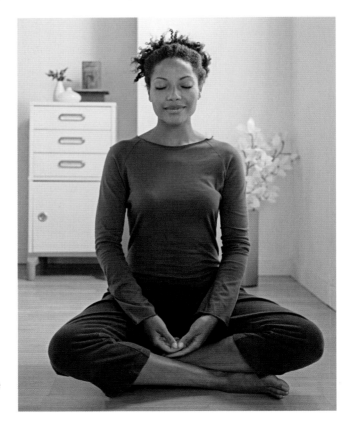

RIGHT: Meditation develops compassion, love and kindness, which help us to help others.

1: Sit comfortably upright, hands resting on knees or thighs. Close your eyes and take your focus inside, watching your breathing slow and lengthen as you become more relaxed. Take your focus to your heart, and look at how you feel now, without analysing.

2: Remember a time when you felt good about yourself. Conjure up the scents and sounds, remember what you were wearing and the room you were in. Let the sensations of happiness, security and inner peace fill you. If you can't remember a specific time, make one up.

Link these feelings with the following phrase, repeating slowly and silently on three exhalations, "May I be happy. May I be well. May I be free from pain." Notice how the words make you feel. If you prefer, make up your own words to express these thoughts.

3: Now think of a good friend. Picture that person in your mind's eye or remember a time you enjoyed together. Let the feelings of love and security you conjured up in step 2 fill your heart. Then send out those feelings, imagining them enveloping your friend, repeating, "May you be perfectly happy. May you be well. May you be free from pain."

4: When you feel ready, think about someone you don't know well. Call up those same feelings, and this time, extend them to that person. Repeat the words. Imagine the recipient enveloped in security and unconditional love.

5: Think of someone you actively dislike; someone who may have caused you pain. Look at the feelings that arise in you when you think about that person. How much happier could you be if you let go of that negativity? See that you have a choice; you don't have to follow those feelings. Now conjure up your happiness scene and let the feelings of love and security erase the uncomfortable feelings. Without thinking too much, send this sentiment out to that person, repeating the phrases. Include yourself, too, if it helps, saying, "May we be perfectly happy…" This has an effect, even if you don't mean it.

6: Finally, bring up the feelings of happiness and peace, and radiate them out to every sentient being in the world. Start with your house, street, town, region, country, continent until you've spread the net of well-wishing as wide as it will stretch. Then sit quietly, adjusting to the room around you.

A long-life community

A good social life and supportive networks keep us in good spirit as we age and prevent cognitive decline and risk of dementia. According to research, social relationships can influence mortality as much as smoking – loneliness is recognized as a first step on the path toward dementia and loss of independent living. The sad news is that if we are socially isolated, we are more likely to die earlier than we might otherwise have done.

We're much more likely to live separately than past generations. In some European countries, more than 40 per cent of women over 65 live alone, according to the WHO. This is a trend even in countries such as Japan that have strong family co-habiting traditions. In the UK, more than half of people live away from their childhood home, and a million over-75s don't know their nearest neighbour.

Community matters more as our nearest depart – losing a partner is a key trigger for withdrawing into the home, risking the social exclusion that contributes to mental and physical decline. Yet life beyond marriage – even if we are widowed – can be long and happy, and choosing to remain living at home alone rather than moving to a care home is associated with greater longevity and better social ties. Loss of a partner for many is a trigger to get out and actively avoid loneliness. In the Longevity Project study (tracking people since the 1920s; see page 361), divorced or widowed women who stayed single were likely to live into their 70s – men required long marriages to make the same age.

More of us now live in "beanpole families", made of several generations but with just a few members of each one. In middle and even old age, we are likely to have both our parents as well as children and adults of various ages around. There's no historical precedent for this, says the WHO. Cross-generational relationships seem to keep us acting young, and increased integration as we age reduces illness – yet the oldest and youngest of us are least likely to be mixing. Around the globe people are fighting such "age apartheid". At Humanitas care home in Deventer in the Netherlands, students live rent-free alongside older people, giving 30 hours per month of service as "good neighbours". Generations cook and shop together, and enjoy the same social activities, from football to partying. Both

RIGHT: By joining in, giving back to our community and sharing time with people of all generations, we make a better space for everyone to grow older in.

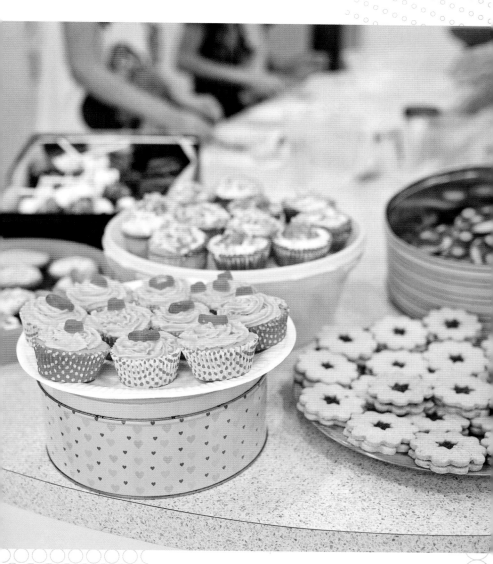

THE SPIRIT OF BABA YAGA

Baba Yaga ("granny witch") is a powerful Russian sorceress with a scary temper and fearsome countenance. She lives in the forest in a hut that stands on hen's feet and is topped with a rooster's head. She eats the disobedient, but those who please her she rewards, and she values resourcefulness most. In Paris, a group of older women has been inspired by her elder energy and set up La Maison des Babayagas (the house of the witches), a self-governing communal housing project where women over 60 live together, with the aim of ageing well, staying active and enjoying being in the centre of things, with the pleasures of city life to hand and life-long learning opportunities (the development encompasses a university for seniors).

In her 1970 treatise on old age, *La Vieillesse*, French writer and feminist Simone de Beauvoir argued that the way in which we regard old age and treat older people exposes a failure in "human civilization". She urged us to rethink every relationship and way of living in order to create a more equitable society. A half-century and millions more old people on, these spirited French feminists taking charge of their own ageing are doing just that.

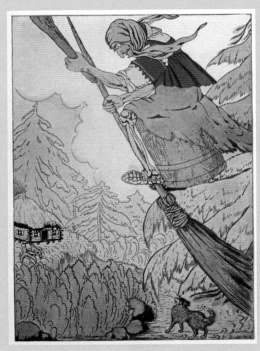

RIGHT: Grandmother witch Baba Yaga most commonly goes riding in a mortar, driving it with a pestle. She sweeps away her trail with a broom of silver birch.

generations seem enthused by the effects. The WHO suggests that older people should be recognized as a resource for younger generations.

Germany has opened 450 multi-generational meeting houses, where everyone can spend time in "public living rooms". Care homes from the UK to Tokyo to Singapore are opening nurseries where activities can be shared, including meals and exercise. Older people benefit from the energy and spirit of the very young, while toddlers soak up the love and experience of elders, breaking down everyone's stereotypes. We don't want segregated activities for the over-50s, research shows. If we're writers, we want writing classes; if we love gardening, we want allotments; if we love music, we want to play in bands, whatever our age.

A report from the International Longevity Centre UK sets out what a community needs for good ageing. More places where all ages can meet and have fun together comes high on the list – playing seems key to healthy ageing – plus cheap and easy ways to get about. A quarter of people over 80 in the UK don't have access to a car, so being able to travel on foot and by bike matters. In the Netherlands, nearly a quarter of journeys made by people over 65 are by bicycle. While we're out socializing we need plenty of places to sit and rest, to eat and use the toilet (lack of public toilets is directly linked with loneliness and isolation – fear strands people at home).

To be part of a community means everyone investing energy to support others. There should be spaces in ageing-friendly towns where people of all ages can share skills and volunteer. When the UK's Royal Institute of British Architects (RIBA) reported on the Third Age in cities, 76 per cent of people over 65 felt that older people had unused wasted talents. The act of helping others seems to reduce depression (one in five people over 65 are estimated to be depressed). In the yoga tradition, community service is a spiritual path all its own – *karma* yoga (selfless service) is a way to self-realization equal in value spiritually to *bhakti* yoga (devotion), *raja* yoga (meditation) and *jnana* yoga (studying sacred texts).

People who immerse themselves in activities and help others tend to live longer – the habit of persistence makes a difference, according to the findings of the Longevity Project (see page 361), having more effect on longevity than a positive outlook or a good sense of humour. Commitment to community service is evident in our involvement in politics as we age. In the US, women over 65 are the demographic most registered to vote, while in the UK, women's share of council seats increases significantly with age; and in local party organization and fundraising it is older women who make a substantial contribution – "I do it because it's right" was a common motivation in a study of older women's activism. Age brings the energy as well as wisdom and compassion for us to say enough is enough, and stand up to change things for the better.

Long-term commitment to a job is also linked with longevity – people who work beyond 55 seem to have a slower loss of cognitive function and live longer than those who retire early, according to a *British Medical Journal* study. Research in a German car plant tracked worker productivity increasing up to age 65.

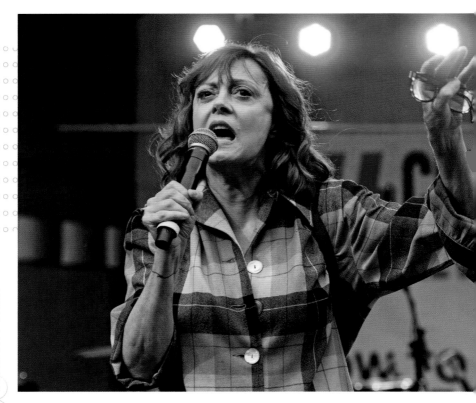

The beneficial effects of work may result from the camaraderie as well as sense of purpose; another study found the more roles we have in life – employee, volunteer, sports club member, parent, sister, congregation member – the better our lung function in older age, and it didn't matter what those roles were.

> "What is more pleasant than old age surrounded by the enthusiasm of youth?"
>
> **CICERO**

LEFT: In 2012, at the age of 66, Susan Sarandon graced the list of Top 10 Celebrity Protesters in *TIME* magazine – living out in her personal life the courageous and outspoken personas she plays on screen.

THE LONGEVITY PROJECT

Psychologists at Stanford University studied the lives of 1,500 people over eight decades, starting in 1921. The plan was to track who lived longest and what psychological factors may have influenced their health and wellbeing. Some of the findings seemed counter-intuitive – marriage didn't seem to safeguard health (divorced women do well), working long hours didn't destroy health (on the contrary, it could lead to longer lives), happiness and an optimistic outlook didn't bring the feel-good benefits we might expect (it led to increased risk-taking, and so death from accidents and smoking). The big lesson was that living in a conscientious way from childhood onward – obeying the rules, keeping on keeping on, valuing prudence and planning, worrying about detail and about not doing the right thing – had a protective role. Persistence made people better at relationships and more embedded in their social networks, more successful at work and more likely to lead a meaningful life filled with purpose. That's the longevity personality.

Healing green and blue

Having access to community green space seems especially useful as we age – in the Nurses' Health Study (of 108,000 women, started in1976 and conducted in the USA), those who had access to most greenness had a 12 per cent lower rate of "all-cause nonaccidental mortality" than those with the least green in their lives. Researchers put it down to reduced risk of depression and increased community engagement.

The opportunity to look out on green space makes us feel comfortable and safe. It reduces stress, anger, frustration and aggression and has a positive effect on mental health and cognitive function, suggest researchers in the Netherlands. Everyone should have access to gardens and parks – and swings and gyms – advises the International Longevity Centre. A pleasant park situated within a ten-minute stroll has an impact on how much we walk, how much time we spend outdoors and how often we are sociable. Outdoor interaction not only makes us perceive our health as better, it strengthens social cohesion in a neighbourhood.

Exposure to water (blue space) has similar effects. The University of Exeter assessed census data from 48 million people in England and

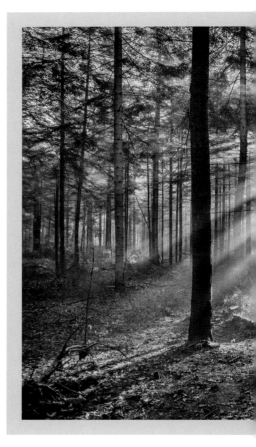

observed that living within reach of the coast correlated with reported better health and happiness. Results were more pronounced in economically deprived communities. Fish tanks have a similar effect – even without fish!

FOREST BATHING

Shinrin-yoku (forest bathing) has been part of Japan's public health system since 1982. People are encouraged to follow woodland therapy trails to benefit from the stress-reducing properties of spending time in nature – basking in natural environments seems to increase blood flow to the brain, and effects on immunity last a month, suggest researchers.

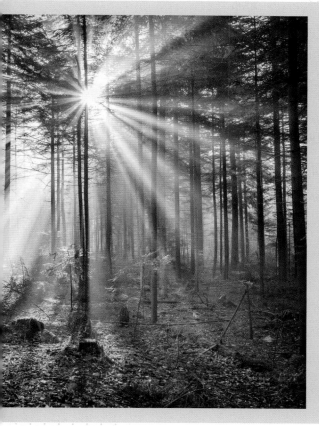

LEFT: Research shows the longer and more frequently we spend time in green spaces, the more active we are and the more benefits we feel for our wellbeing and mental health.

"It is not so much for its beauty that the forest makes a claim upon men's hearts, as for that subtle something, that quality of the air, that emanation from the old trees, that so wonderfully changes and renews a weary spirit."

ROBERT LOUIS STEVENSON

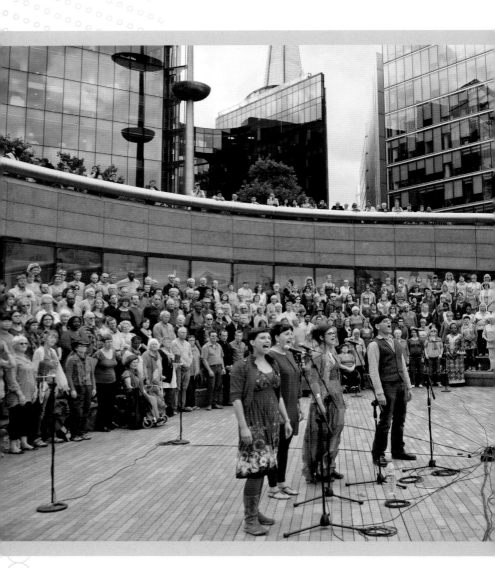

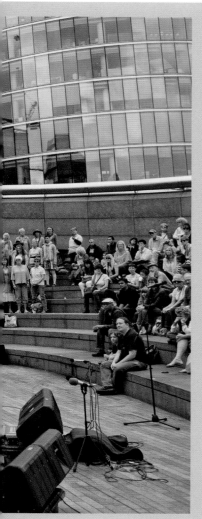

THE SPIRIT OF SONG

There are measurable health benefits to joining a community choir as we get older, says the UK's National Institute for Health and Care Excellence (NICE). As well as social benefits – counteracting loneliness and depression, keeping us active and providing a good reason to get out of the house – choral singing seems to build lower-body strength and balance and aid memory and executive function (the mental capacity to plan, organize and get things done) while reducing stress and promoting feel-good endorphins. It's linked with fewer visits to the doctor and less use of medicine. Other community-based arts projects studied for their energizing health effects include creative writing and art classes, but choirs give back, too. They bring pleasure to audiences and transmit cultural heritage. Choirs root us to a place and help us express that connection as we send feelings on the wing of song out beyond our lives and into the future.

In yoga terms, singing activates *vishuddha*, the throat chakra, the energy centre connected with empathy and tuning in to the vibrations of others. It's from here that we express our creativity and stand up for ourselves to communicate what we need to be happy. When this energy centre functions well, it is said to lead to long life.

LEFT: Our heart rates sync when we sing as a group – and a 2008 study by Harvard and Yale Universities found that choral singing increased life expectancy.

Fruit of the earth

Gardening not only boosts cardiovascular health; growing things also encourages habits associated with mental and emotional wellbeing, such as self-esteem and persistence. The more sedentary, solitary and indoors we are, the greater the benefits of taking up gardening. In studies, people were more likely to keep up gardening than a gym regime, and the continuity of the routine and ritual promoted memory. Allotment gardening seems particularly beneficial – its semi-public nature enhances social and cultural integration and combats isolation.

There's comfort in the thought that, as we grow older and spend more time in one place, we are what we eat – our bodies become part of a place, if we eat the produce of that soil and climate and geology, or *terroir*. Bone-testing on ancient skeletons can pinpoint where those people grew up, their surroundings literally infused in their bones. If we take the time and trouble to find out what grows well in our particular soil and climate, and raise plants that have a long history in our area, that helps us ingest our culture and landscape and express our identity. As we get older and

RIGHT: When we raise plants and cultivate a garden, we become aware at a very physical level of time passing and of death leading to new growth. This can feel grounding and healing.

perception of time passing quickens, so the cycle of tilling, sowing, transplanting, nurturing, harvesting and eating becomes more perceptible. What better way to gain pleasure from the passage of time? Cicero, writing about old age, referred to

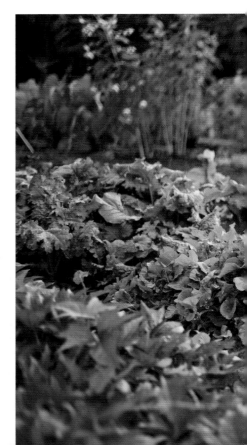

the pleasure of watching grapes on the vine bud and swell, the moisture of the earth and warmth of the sun nourishing them from bitterness to sweet maturity. There's a metaphorical lesson on the sweetness of life coming to fruition.

> *"Your descendants shall gather your fruits."*
>
> **VIRGIL**

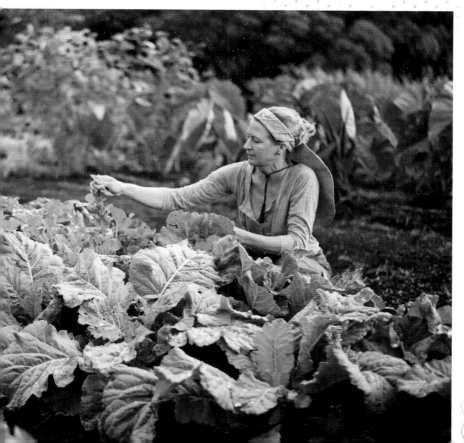

IMPROVISED WARM-UPS

Trust exercises are useful ice-breakers in cross-generational creative groups. These drama and stand-up warm-ups offer playful ideas to explore.

- **Share the move** Stand in a circle. One person starts moving a part of the body (toe, finger, nose), starting small and making the movement bigger until they "throw" the move to someone else at random, who continues it. The second person develops the move, taking it into another part of the body and, when ready, throws it to someone else. This stimulates eye contact while loosening the body and imagination.

- **Sit, stand, lean** Take three people: one sits, one stands, one leans. Now put yourselves in a situation – at the doctor's, on the sports field, in the classroom – and improvise a scene. Change position as you improvise, making sure someone is always sitting, standing and leaning.

I bow to you

Namaste – the traditional Indian greeting, spoken with palms together at the heart – translates as "the divine in me bows to the divine in you", alluding to the belief that a spark of divine lives in all of us, within the heart. By bringing our palms together at the centre of the chest (a hand position known as *Anjali Mudra*) we honour this connection to others. The pressure in the palms activates minor chakras that connect with the heart, while bringing together right and left hand stimulates both sides of the brain.

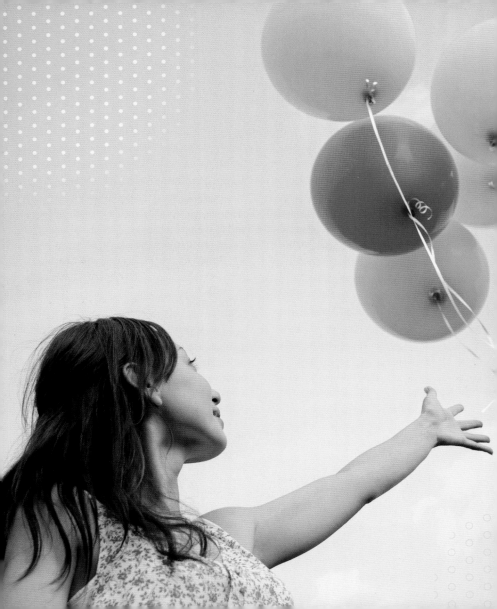

A life's journey

Age brings all manner of vulnerabilities, anxiety and feelings of fragility as mind, body and family life seem to crumble along with our position in society. We can feel empty, like we've lost the potential people we could have been.

Perhaps there are fewer reference points for what we'll be in the future. Forced change of circumstance, disquieting uncertainty and saying goodbye to parts of ourselves are all hard on the spirit.

On the other hand, ageing also offers the opportunity to let go of stuff that no longer serves us – things we didn't manage to achieve, expectations we didn't meet – to make room for different things. Once children leave home, jobs close down, hormones decline and we've spent time honouring the grief, finding our bearings and regrouping, then there is space to nurture new things that require our generous time and attention, maybe a creative practice or a business, a new place to live or fresh passion. Carl Jung described life as having a morning, afternoon and evening, and explained that the activities that might suit life's morning may not be appropriate for its afternoons or evenings. Each programme of activity has its own time, and as we pass through the day we find just as much meaning and purpose in the new things appropriate for each time slot. If we dwell on morning concerns in the evening, we will not thrive.

Cocooning is a useful spiritual practice at times of transition. When we feel wobbly on the outside, turning inside with meditation techniques helps us adjust expectations and test out new aspects of ourselves in safety. Then when we reach a fork in the road, we can choose a new path, using the experience, practical lessons and compassion gained over decades to make illusion-free decisions about what next, to see there has been purpose to life so far, and plenty more to come.

LEFT: Daring to let go can be a liberating and exhilarating experience that makes space for new life.

Containment

1. Rest in Child's Pose (*Balasana*, see page 65), with or without supports. This is a position of surrender and worship that puts the forehead in touch with the energy of the earth, for deep tranquillity. We can rest here and wait for the universe to do its thing.

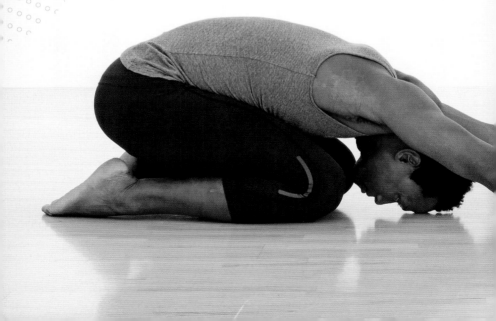

2. Bring your attention to the way your breath moves your back. Feel it expanding around your sacrum and widening your back ribs. Contemplate the precious life force, *prana*, in each breath and feel it riding in and out. The front of the body in yoga represents the individual – it's where our sense organs are. The back of the body represents community – everything else in the universe. We usually neglect it because our senses keep us focused forward. The back of the body in yoga is also considered the west side, soft and yielding to the east's activating energy. Think about the energy of the sun rising in the east and setting in the west. Allow the energy of the west and the connection to the universe to help you adjust to what is to come. In forward bending we surrender to the forces of nature at work in ageing, while feeling safely cocooned.

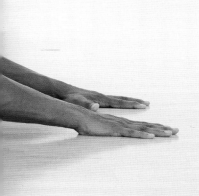

Instant reassurance

Placing a soft weight over the forehead brings instant calm and a sense of being kind to yourself. It depresses the neurovascular points on the forehead – in the same way that on hearing bad news we might place a palm over the forehead, an instinctive human reaction.

• Rest in Corpse Pose (*Savasana*, see page 385) and place a folded towel or eye pillow over your forehead for eight minutes or longer. In Iyengar Yoga we might wrap a long crepe bandage around the head (not too tightly) before relaxing, which feels incredibly reassuring.

RETHINKING WHO WE ARE

On the journey of ageing it's useful to take time to reconsider where and who we are as circumstances change – to ask if life is still meaningful and happy. The following questions can nurture an inner life and sense of spirituality that helps us withstand negative emotions, such as vulnerability and grief, and cultivate hope and a self-sufficient sense of purpose:

• What has been my life purpose to this point?
• What might it be now?
• What makes me feel whole?
• Which experiences are worth taking forward?
• What loose ends could I tie up?
• Are my relationships satisfying?
• How can I find new forms of intimacy and connection?
• What did contentment mean to me?
• What makes life worth living now?
• What's hard right now?
• How do I cope with tough stuff?
• Do I have a framework for hope – is that from a spiritual tradition?
• Am I more able than I was to live with ambiguity and uncertainty?

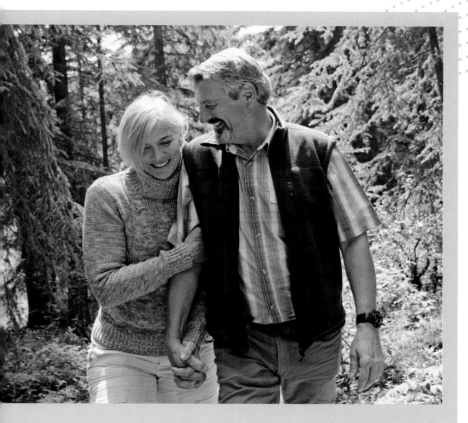

- What's left undone or unsaid – can I do anything about that?
- How have I made the world a better place?
- What was the value of my life?
- What will live on – what's my legacy?

ABOVE: Take regular time out from the weekly routine to consider what's really important, rethink priorities and renegotiate relationships.

Time meditation

The body is constantly evolving, which is obvious in some life stages – babyhood, adolescence, pregnancy, menopause – but cells are always dying and renewing. There is no set body. This meditation brings the empowering awareness that we are not the physical body but a constant "me" within.

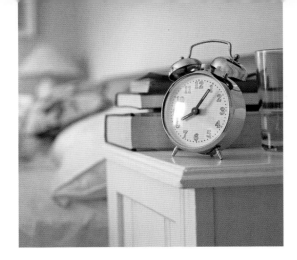

1. Sit or kneel comfortably, hands resting on knees or thighs. Close your eyes and focus your mind by watching the waves of breath moving in and out.

2. When your mind feels tranquil, start to ponder your body. Imagine the midline of your emerging spine, days after conception; see your fingers and toes when you were newborn; visualize your arms and legs as a two-year-old and as an eight-year-old; think about the changes of adolescence; if you are a mother, remember the physical changes of pregnancy. Understand that the body is constantly in flux; it does not define who you are.

3. Start to watch your mind. See it as a blank screen and watch thoughts projected on it without engaging with them. See how you remain at one remove from your thoughts. They are not you.

4. Next notice sensations – pins and needles in your legs perhaps, an itchy nose, an urge to sneeze, air on bare skin. See how the sensations change as time passes, and understand that stimulation of the sense receptors is separate from you.

5. Appreciate the freedom of not having to be your body, thoughts or sensations. Relish the potential this represents. Use the knowledge to help you decide what you want from life and to set in action the changes to bring it about.

Five acts of life

The human brain is primed to find meaning. Given a random set of events, we can't resist introducing cause and effect to turn it into a story. This is helpful as we get older and strive to pin down meanings of life. Working on a life story that emphasizes spirituality helps people develop stronger relationships with other people and staff in care homes. This exercise uses story-structure techniques to help make sense of life so far and yet to come. Use the prompts to write your life story in five acts.

Act 1: Who are you and what's your emotional state? What's your goal? Why do people care about you? What gets you started on your life's journey?

Act 2: What reluctance do you have following this path? What obstacles do you face? Do you gain knowledge and how does this change you or your goal?

Act 3: What do you learn in the middle of your story that changes the way you see life or your goal? What happens if you don't change? What's your emotional state in the middle of your story?

Act 4: What doubts do you experience? What is your greatest obstacle to achieving your goal – and how do you confront that, and change?

Act 5: Do you achieve your goal? Or do you choose another path? Do you discover your true self or higher purpose? What is your emotional state at the end of your story? Why do people care about you now?

Energy of change

Kali is the fierce Hindu goddess who offers strength at times of change. She is the spirit of time and embodies its cycles, the changes they bring and all the terrifying powers of time to create and destroy. Dark blue with three staring eyes and tongue poking out, she is depicted trampling the dead body of her husband Siva. Around her waist hangs a belt of skulls and a fringe of human hands, while she brandishes a severed head dripping blood from one of her four hands, a chopper in another. The intensity of her annihilating energy is terrifying. She's intoxicated by it as she faces her enemies and battles demons. She is the most awe-ful of the Hindu representations of divine energy, and depicts how life can feel in this stage – raw, bloody, world-ending.

But Kali's remaining two hands offer blessings and in India she is worshipped as the Divine Mother whose fierce energy gives us the power to stand up to the very worst and emerge with energy and spirit intact. After the death of everything comes new growth and Kali signposts our endless creative potential.

RIGHT: The Hindu goddess Kali is terrifying – staring at her should jolt us out of our everyday thinking. She emboldens us if we can channel some of that raw power.

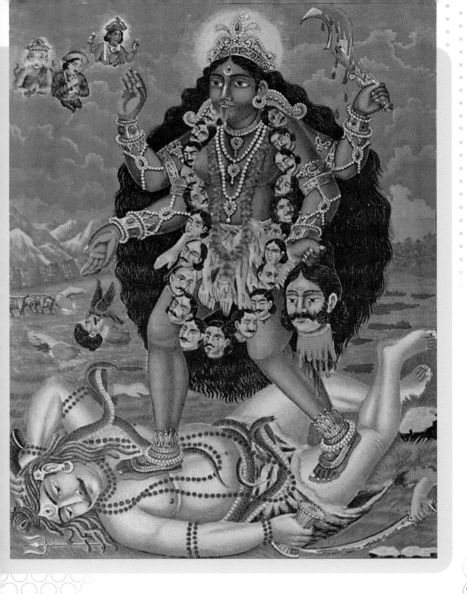

Kali pose

This simple standing position fills us with the fierce creative energy of Kali and feels incredibly potent.

1. Stand in horse stance, feet wider than hip-width apart and turning out a little, knees slightly bent. Rest your hands on your hips.

2. As you exhale, bend into a deeper squat and raise your arms, elbows bent in a 90-degree cactus shape and fingers spread, palms facing forward. Breathe out audibly through your mouth, "haaaaa". Stick out your tongue if it feels good.

3. As you inhale, come back to horse stance. Repeat the squat and sounded out-breath another four to six times. Look forward and feel the fierce energy of Kali in the strength of your legs and your powerful upper body.

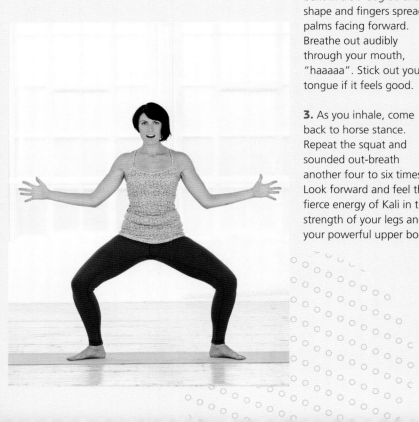

Impermanence contemplation

This exercise is a qigong warm-up. Walk five paces in any direction, stop and watch the body being still. When you feel ready, take another five paces in any direction and stop again. Repeat for five minutes in total, moving where the impulse takes you and stopping for as long as you feel necessary. There's no need to make the paces a single length, or to walk forward – try sideways, diagonal, backward, tiny steps or longer strides. Notice how awareness of impermanence is strangely grounding.

Doing a deal with death

Myths contain great wisdom. They're our way of exploring and articulating the deepest, and often most unpalatable, truths of what it is to be human. In many traditions, we find stories of the forfeit we must pay for coming back to life after entering the underworld. Greek goddess of fertility Persephone is abducted by Hades, ruler of the underworld, and forced to become queen of his dominion. Eventually, she is restored to the upper world and life, but since she has consumed pomegranate seeds down below, she is compelled to return there, spending a third of each year away from the fertile earth. If you've had a life-altering illness, what's your own deal, what do you give up in order to go back to your old world? It might be to quit smoking, know you can't put on weight, stick to an exercise regime. Contemplate the ways in which your body and mind have been altered completely by this event, and what new kind of human being you've become.

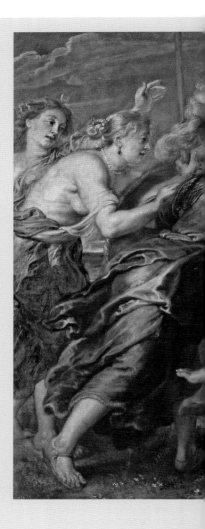

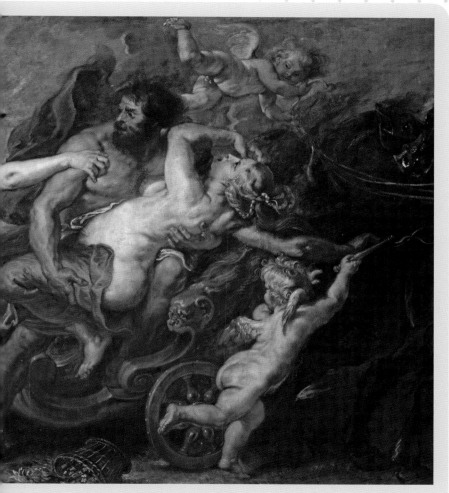

ABOVE: The abduction of Persephone by the god of the underworld, as seen by Rubens. She must become both queen of the dead and the bringer of new life after winter.

The qualities of winter

In art, winter is depicted as an old woman; we might think of her as a grandmother spirit or wise old crone. Hers is a welcome quiet time after the energy and activity of summer and fruiting of autumn, a time to draw in, rest and reflect after the full and active months. An endless summer would be depleting, flowers constantly open would not fruit and the plant would not conserve enough energy to pass on its seed. Winter is necessary in the cycle of the year, the time we gather in and save seeds – kernels with the capacity for new life and many happy returns of the year. We might not see all the plants that grow from these seeds, but we gain strength from their power and potential, the creative energy sealed in the pods.

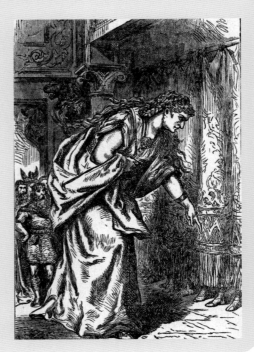

RIGHT: Skadi, Norse goddess of winter and hunting, choosing her husband Njord (the one with the most beautiful feet, concealed behind the curtain). She is a giant in the room.

Corpse pose

At the end of every yoga class comes relaxation in Corpse Pose (*Savasana*). In its stillness, without movement of body or mind, we imitate death. It's a difficult pose, yet we long for its nothingness throughout class, for the letting go that leads to deep restoration and rejuvenation.

1. Lie on your back – relax your arms away from your body, palms up. Curl your shoulders beneath you to open your armpits, important energy centres. Stretch your legs away comfortably, wide enough apart to release the lower back. Let your feet flop outward.

2. Feel the ground supporting the full weight of your pelvis, the back of your head, your shoulders and heels. Sink downward.

3. Have an image of yourself heavy on the earth, dropping down and becoming the earth, nourishing the soil so that trees grow out of you, absorb the carbon dioxide the world exhales and send out new oxygen. You are part of the earth and the tree and the air. You are the molecules that make up everything in the universe.

4. When ready, feel the world around you. Imagine its colours. Feel the sensation of air on your face. Slowly move your fingers and toes and tongue. Stretch, then roll to one side before pushing up to sit.

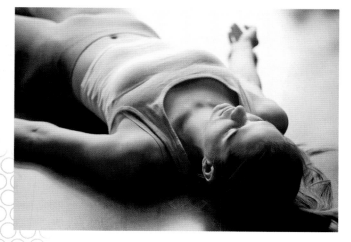

End of sound awareness

A sound meditation is a useful introduction to endings. It may seem perverse, but contemplating death jolts us into awareness of the present, so we appreciate and make the most of every minute. For this exercise, you'll need a bell or cymbal.

Sit quietly, close your eyes and sound a bell or chime a cymbal. Follow the sound waves as they change; notice how the pureness of the initial sound becomes richer and more resonant as the sound lengthens, then becomes most engrossing for the ear as it fades to imperceptible waves. Tune in to the four stages of sound – the silence from which it emerges, the beginning of the sound, its sustenance, then decline and return to silence. Nothingness, growth, sustenance, decline into nothingness – a metaphor for the human condition.

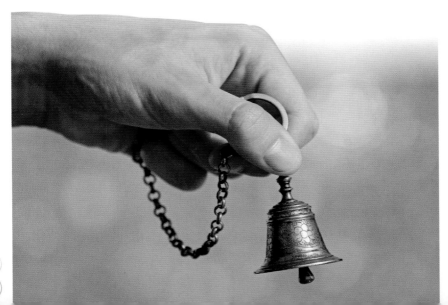

Breath-retention contemplation

This is another way to contemplate endings and appreciate the silence, space and feeling of the endless opportunities they bring. As you practise, ask if there's anything you'd like to cease doing. If you feel breathless or stressed, return to your normal breath pattern.

1. Sit comfortably upright and follow your breathing. After a while, watch the gaps at the end of the out-breath before you inhale, and at the top of the in-breath, before you start to breathe out.

2. At the end of your next in-breath can you retain the breath for a little (without straining)? At the end of the out-breath hold that pause, too, for a bit.

3. Repeat, pausing at the end of each in- and out-breath and extending the length of time you hold them. Can you sense the difference between the nothingness of the in- and out-breath? How does it feel just to stop? Enjoy having nothing to do. Feel the potential in stopping. Continue for as long as you can maintain focus, then return to your regular breathing pattern.

"The self is not born, it dies not. It sprang from nothing, nothing sprang from it. The ancient is unborn, eternal, everlasting; he is not killed, though the body is killed."

**KATHA UPANISHAD,
ANCIENT SANSKRIT PHILOSOPHICAL TEXT**

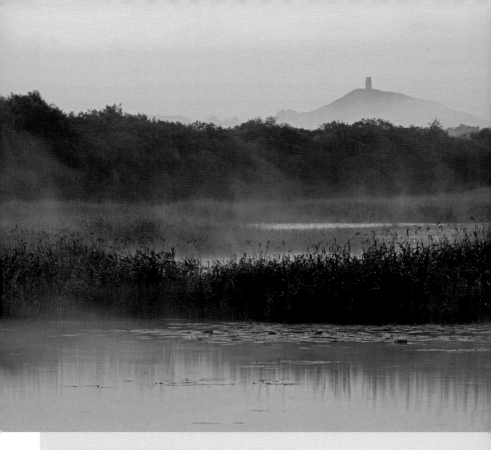

Island of life ever after

In the far far west, at the point where the sun sets into the sea at the end of the day, lies the Isle of Avalon, the place where the wounded King Arthur is guided by the Lady of the Lake after his last battle. Dante, like Cicero, writes of old age as a peaceful navigation home. We sight land and coast

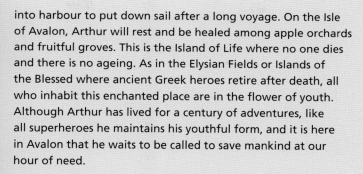

into harbour to put down sail after a long voyage. On the Isle of Avalon, Arthur will rest and be healed among apple orchards and fruitful groves. This is the Island of Life where no one dies and there is no ageing. As in the Elysian Fields or Islands of the Blessed where ancient Greek heroes retire after death, all who inhabit this enchanted place are in the flower of youth. Although Arthur has lived for a century of adventures, like all superheroes he maintains his youthful form, and it is here in Avalon that he waits to be called to save mankind at our hour of need.

Chinese mythology tells of Islands of the Blest, "spirit mountains" set in the ocean but impossible to find because they are shrouded, like Avalon, in mist and sink beneath the waves when mortals venture close. There is a fountain of youthful vigour here, among the precious jewels and herbs of everlasting life. As with Avalon, explorers have set out to find these islands, but the only sure way to navigate to them is through magical practices, *fangshi*, that preserve body and mind.

Some suggest these islands correspond to the longevity lands of Okinawa, and Japanese tales echo their mountainous form and tree of life hung with jewels and moss of immortality. Perpetual life in one Japanese tale is something the island's inhabitants find so distressing that they long for the mortal condition. We learn that immortality is only for the divine – and superheroes such as Arthur. For us mortals it will always be just out of reach; our best hope of immortality is the legacy of a life well lived.

LONGEVITY SPIRIT

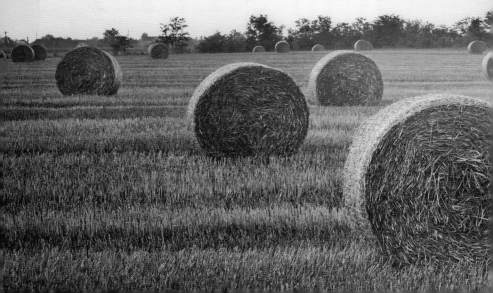

"Now the harvest of old age is, as I have often said, the memory and rich store of blessings laid up in easier life. Again, all things that accord with nature are to be counted as good. But what can be more in accordance with Nature than for old men to die?... old men die like a fire going out because it has burnt down of its own nature without artificial means. Again, just as apples when unripe are torn from trees, but when ripe and mellow drop down, so it is violence that takes life from young men, ripeness from old. This ripeness is so delightful to me that, as I approach nearer to death, I seem, as it were, to be sighting land, and to be coming to port at last after a long voyage."

CICERO

Recommended reading

Allen, Katherine, *The Qigong Bible,* Godsfield Press, 2017

Aurelius, Marcus, *Meditations*, Penguin Classics, 2006

Barnes, Julian, *The Sense of an Ending,* Vintage, 2012

de Beauvoir, Simone, *The Coming of Age*, W. W. Norton & Company, 1996

Bolen, Jean Shinoda, *Goddesses in Older Women*, HarperCollins, 2014

Brown, Christina, *The Modern Yoga Bible*, Godsfield Press, 2017

Cicero, *On Living and Dying Well*, Penguin Classics, 2012

Colette, *Break of Day*, Farrar, Straus and Giroux, 2002

Collard, Patrizia, *The Mindfulness Bible*, Godsfield Press , 2015

Dickinson, Emily, *The Complete Poems,* Faber & Faber, 2016

Dinsmore-Tuli, Uma, *Yoni Shakti,* YogaWords, 2014

Docherty, Dan, *The Tai Chi Bible*, Godsfield Press, 2014

Estés, Clarissa Pinkola, *Women Who Run With the Wolves,* Rider, 2008

Forster, E.M., *Aspects of the Novel*, Penguin Classics, 2005

Graves, Robert, *The Greek Myths*, Penguin, 2017

Iyengar, B.K.S., *Yoga: The Path to Holistic Health*, DK, 2014

Jung, C.G. (introduced by Anthony Storr), *The Essential Jung*, Fontana Press, 1998

Kneipp, Sebastian, *My Water-Cure*, Forgotten Books, 2017

Lad, Vasant, *The Complete Book of Ayurvedic Home Remedies*, Piatkus, 2006

Lively, Penelope, *Ammonites & Leaping Fish*, Penguin, 2014

Long, Diane and Hoare, Sophy, *Notes on Yoga, The Legacy of Vanda Scaravelli,* YogaWords, 2017

Marlowe, Christopher, *Doctor Faustus*, Longman, 2003

Marriott, Susannah, *Witches, Sirens and Soothsayers*, Spruce, 2008

Myers, Thomas W, *Anatomy Trains: Myofascial Meridians for Manual and Movement Therapists*, Churchill Livingstone, 2013

Pilates, Joseph H. and Miller, William J., *Return to Life Through Contrology*, Martino Fine Books, 2014

Rice, Sam and Spencer, Mimi, *The Midlife Kitchen*, Mitchell Beazley, 2017

Robinson, Marilynne, *Lila*, Virago, 2014

Saradananda, Swami, *Chakra Meditation*, Duncan Baird Publishers, 2011

Saradananda, Swami, *The Power of Breath*, Watkins, 2017

Sarton, May, *Plant Dreaming Deep*, W. W. Norton & Company, 1996

Semlyen, Anne and Trewhela, Alison, *Yoga for Healthy Lower Backs*, Lotus Publishing, 2011

Shakespeare, William, *King Lear,* Oxford University Press, 2008

Shakespeare, William, *The Winter's Tale,* Oxford University Press, 2008

Small, Helen, *The Long Life*, Oxford University Press, 2010

Townsend Warner, Sylvia, *Lolly Willowes*, Virago, 2012

Vogler, Christopher, *The Writer's Journey: Mythic Structure for Writers,* Michael Wiese Productions, 2007

Yorke, John, *Into the Woods*, Penguin, 2014

Online Resources

Introduction to Therapeutic and Reflective Writing, www.profwritingacademy.com/therapeutic-and-reflective-writing

Index

Acknowledgements

Special thanks to Leanne, for her brilliant ideas and for getting the ball rolling, and to Ella and the Octopus team. I'd like to thank my yoga teacher Amanda Brown for 12 years of twice-weekly inspiration, and all the other fantastic ageing role models in my life, but especially Christina Bunce, Helen Shipman, Jane Pugh, Mary Mathieson, Lyn Gardner and Jo Leevers. Thanks to Gill Garrett for stoic thoughts and Dan Cadwallader for the Hammer take on ageing.

Picture Credits

akg-images Peter Connolly 315. **Alamy Stock Photo** Anna Ivanova 213; ART Collection 379; Art Collection 2 335; Art Collection 4 151; Chronicle 108, 288, 358; Dinodia Photos 99; Lebrecht Music and Arts Photo Library 219; Michael Kemp 364; Mustafa Ismail 208; Olga Miltsova 246; Paul Fearn 384; Science Photo Library 71; Stefan Dahl Langstrup 60; Stephen Spraggon 388; Tim Gainey 20; Wavebreak Media Ltd. 147; Westend61 GmbH 10. **Bridgeman Images** Birmingham Museums and Art Gallery 268; J. Paul Getty Museum, Los Angeles, USA 25; Pictures from History 305. **Dreamstime.com** Anna Bocharova 35; Natalia Bachkova 322; Petr Goskov 233; Tilltibet 19; Wabeno 187; Wavebreakmedia Ltd. 18. **Getty Images** A. Chederros 239; Alistair Berg 333; Andrea Wyner 117; Ascent/PKS Media Inc. 84; Ben Welsh 327; Blend Images – KidStock 45; BLOOM image 370; Bloom Productions 266; BSIP/UIG 101; David Lees 34; David McLain 351; DEA/G. CIGOLINI/Contributor 29; Dean Conger/Corbis via Getty Images 179; Dimitri Otis 160; Dominik Ketz/Contributor 338; Dougal Waters 36, 163, 376; Eric Fougere/Sygma via Getty Images 13b; Fancy/Veer/Corbis 252; Fine Art Images/Heritage Images 382; GARO 343; Hero Images 47, 295, 348, 375; Jamie Grill 46; Jose A. Bernat Bacete 386; Jose Luis Pelaez Inc. 347; Jupiterimages 336; Kjell Linder 366; Leemage/Corbis via Getty Images 39; Pascal Parrot/Sygma/Sygma via Getty Images 13a; Photo12/UIG via Getty Images 30; Rob Lewine 354; stilllifephotographer 323; Tetra Images 37; Thierry Dosogne 313; Westend61 7, 10; ZenShui/Frederic Cirou 285; Zu Sanchez Photography 26. **iStock** 4kodiak 204; andresr 205; AntiMartina 241; anyaberkut 303; Avalon_Studio 189; Aviator70 283; bee32 261; Creativeye99 202; darjeelingsue 231; den-belitsky 236; dogfeeder 192; el_clicks 357; eurobanks 201; FatCamera 43, 59, 274; fcafotodigital 190; fizkes 125, 385; GCShutter 145; GMVozd 330; gnagel 321; GoodLifeStudio 299; graphicgeoff 220; gregory_lee 235; id-art 182; illustrart 186; jeffbergen 106; jenifoto 215; JensGade 191; Johnny Greig 223; juliedeshaies 193; konradlew 8, 362; kupicoo 218; laflor 301; Lecic 188; Magone 194; MarcoRof 111; monkeybusinessimages 184; mthipsorn 318; nerudol 195; Neustockimages 142, 324; OksanaKiian 210; ooyoo 248; Parshina Olga 69; PeopleImages 118, 264, 272, 296, 310; Rastan 352; rezkrr 249; Sasha_Suzi 58; scisettialfio 245; seanrmcdermid 199; SelectStock 140; splendens 308; spooh 316; Thomas_Zsebok_Images 390; vgajic 56; voinSveta 17; Wavebreakmedia Ltd. 312; YakubovAlim 198; YelenaYemchuk 259; YinYang 197; zeljkosantrac 216; ZU_09 77. **J. Paul Getty Museum** 176. **Metropolitan Museum of Art** Bequest of Phyllis Massar, 2011 250; The Elisha Whittelsey Collection, The Elisha Whittelsey Fund, 1951 28. **Octopus Publishing Group** Ian Wallace 255; Russell Sadur 126, 229; Ruth Jenkinson 40, 49, 52, 62, 64, 68, 73, 74, 80a, 82, 83, 88, 90, 92, 95, 103, 113, 114, 119, 120, 122, 129, 130, 131, 133, 136, 139, 153, 154, 165, 168, 172, 174, 224, 226, 276, 280, 290, 340, 344, 369, 372, 380, 381; William Shaw 256, 257. **Pixabay** Pitsch 242; urformat 104. **Press Association Images** NurPhoto/SIPA USA 360. **Science Photo Library** Dr. P. Marazzi 265; Gwen Shockey 14; Mauro Fermariello 51; Nicolle R. Fuller 287; Sovereign/ISM 270. **Shutterstock** Brian A Jackson 23; Gekko Gallery 278. **SuperStock** Fine Art Photographic Library 158; Lucenet Patrice/Oredia Eurl 171. **Wellcome Collection** 207.